FUNDAMENTALS OF HEMATOLOGY

INTERNAL MEDICINE SERIES

Coordinating Editors

JACK D. MYERS, M.D.
University Professor of Medicine, University of Pittsburgh

DAVID E. ROGERS, M.D.
President, The Robert Wood Johnson Foundation
Princeton, New Jersey

RESPIRATORY INSUFFICIENCY
Benjamin Burrows, M.D., Ronald J. Knudson, M.D.
and Louis J. Kettel, M.D.

ENDOCRINE DISORDERS: A Pathophysiologic Approach
Will G. Ryan, M.D.

GASTROINTESTINAL DISORDERS: A Pathophysiologic Approach
Norton J. Greenberger, M.D. and Daniel H. Winship, M.D.

FUNDAMENTALS OF HEMATOLOGY
Richard A. Rifkind, M.D., Arthur Bank, M.D.,
Paul A. Marks, M.D. and Hymie L. Nossel, M.D.

Fundamentals of Hematology

by

RICHARD A. RIFKIND, M.D.

Professor of Medicine and Human Genetics and Development,
Columbia University, College of Physicians & Surgeons;
Director, Hematology Division and Training Program,
Columbia-Presbyterian Medical Center, New York

ARTHUR BANK, M.D.

Professor of Medicine and Human Genetics and Development,
Columbia University, College of Physicians & Surgeons;
Chief, Leukemia-Lymphoma Study Group,
Columbia-Presbyterian Medical Center, New York

PAUL A. MARKS, M.D.

Frode Jensen Professor of Medicine and
Professor of Human Genetics and Development,
Columbia University, College of Physicians & Surgeons;
Director, Cancer Research Center,
Columbia-Presbyterian Medical Center, New York

HYMIE L. NOSSEL, M.D.

Professor of Medicine,
Columbia University,
College of Physicians & Surgeons;
Chief, Hemostasis Study Group and Laboratories,
Columbia-Presbyterian Medical Center, New York

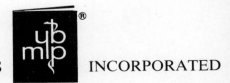

YEAR BOOK MEDICAL PUBLISHERS INCORPORATED

35 EAST WACKER DRIVE / CHICAGO

Library of Congress Catalog Card Number: 76-3146

International Standard Book Number: 0-8151-7335-0

Preface

THE PURPOSE of this book is to provide, in a relatively concise manner, a body of knowledge that can serve students interested in exploring hematology as well as physicians seeking a reliable but concise review of hematologic problems. The material represents our current understanding of the biologic basis of hematology and the basis of clinical practice. Indeed, the present text is derived in part from a syllabus that has been used, with many revisions, over the past 10 years at the College of Physicians and Surgeons of Columbia University. The volume of material presented has been held in check by selecting areas of importance without sacrificing sophistication or accuracy. The text is not documented by citations to the literature. Instead, those seeking to explore further any of the problems developed are referred to the several major encyclopedic textbooks presently available and to the several excellent reviews of topics in hematology. A list of recommended readings appears at the end of the text. All sections of this book are provided with numerical indices, which permits the reader to refer easily to other pertinent sections. While the authors collectively accept full responsibility for any defects in this textbook, the major responsibilities were divided as follows: hematopoietic development (P.A.M.), red cell disorders (R.A.R.), white cell disorders (A.B.) and hemostasis (H.L.N.).

One cautionary note, none of the "facts" provided in this text are immutable; rather, they represent our present best judgment. We have tried to indicate where the evidence is strong and where it is weak. Ultimately, the very process of re-evaluation and revision is the only truly immutable aspect of medical science.

RICHARD A. RIFKIND
ARTHUR BANK
PAUL A. MARKS
HYMIE L. NOSSEL

Table of Contents

1

Developmental Aspects of Hematopoiesis

1.1 Introduction

CELLULAR PROLIFERATION, differentiation, morphogenesis, functional maturation and senescence constitute the basic patterns of hematopoiesis. The hematopoietic tissues and clinical hematology have proved uniquely valuable as a model for a cell biology-oriented approach to human pathophysiology. For this reason it is valuable to begin our study with an analysis of the developmental history of hematopoietic cells, their origins during embryogenesis and the nature of the regulatory mechanisms that control proliferation and differentiation in response to body needs. In later chapters the implications of these fundamental patterns for a variety of clinical problems in hematology will be explored in detail.

The process of embryogenesis and cell differentiation in animals, including man, involves a remarkably ordered program of changes. A variety of morphologic and functional changes occur simultaneously and sequentially in a developing organism. The mechanisms determining and controlling these processes remain one of the major unsolved problems in biology. A great deal of what we do understand about the differentiation of eukaryotic cells, the genetic control of expression of specialized functions and the sequential events at organismal, cellular and organellar levels that characterize development and differentiation has been learned from a study of hematopoietic cell systems in both man and experimental animals.

In this context hematopoiesis may be considered with respect to the following aspects:

1. Organ sites of hematopoiesis in the developing fetus, the newborn infant and adult human subjects.

2. Relationship between primitive and definitive hematopoietic cell lines.

1

3. Patterns of hemoglobin synthesis during fetal development and in adult life.

4. Regulation of hematopoiesis.

1.2 Organ Sites of Hematopoiesis during Fetal Development

The first detectable sites of hematopoiesis during human fetal development are the blood islands of the yolk sac, which are detectable at approximately 19–20 days of gestation (Fig. 1–1). It is generally believed that these blood islands are derived from the mesodermal extraembryonic cell layer of the yolk sac, although there is evidence that the endoderm also may play a contributory role in organizing hematopoiesis. The blood islands are an active site of hematopoiesis only through the eighth to 12th weeks of gestation. The yolk sac blood islands are largely erythropoietic (red cell-producing) organs, but there is evidence that granulocyte and megakaryocyte precursors also are present during this stage of hematopoiesis. Morpho-

Fig. 1–1.—Sites of hematopoiesis during human fetal development and the sequence of appearance of formed blood elements in the circulation. *Broken lines* indicate that the precise timing is not established. The yolk sac is the site of primitive erythroid cell development. The liver, spleen and bone marrow are all sites of production of definitive erythroid cells.

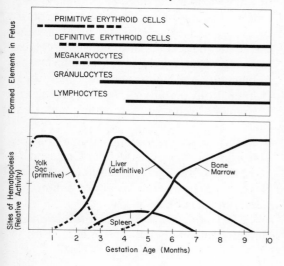

logically identifiable hematopoiesis begins within the fetus proper in the liver during the fifth to sixth weeks of gestation. The fetal liver becomes and remains the primary site of hematopoiesis until the sixth month of gestation and may continue to produce blood cells in normal subjects until about 1–2 weeks after birth. Initially the hematopoietic cells of the fetal liver are almost entirely erythroid. Granulocytopoiesis begins in the fetal liver but is not prominent until the onset of hematopoiesis in the bone marrow. The spleen is a site of hematopoiesis during fetal life between the fourth and the eighth months of gestation. The bone marrow becomes the principal site of hematopoiesis after the sixth month of gestation. After 3 weeks of age (post partum), under normal conditions the bone marrow becomes the only active site of hematopoiesis and remains active throughout childhood and adult life.

1.3 Primitive and Definitive Hematopoietic Cell Lineages

The erythroid cells produced by the yolk sac blood islands are unique in their pattern of morphogenesis and in the hemoglobins they produce. Since this cell line is transient and limited to early embryogenesis, it is referred to as the primitive hematopoietic cell lineage. Morphologically these cells are characterized by their large size and by the fact that the mature primitive erythrocyte fails to extrude its nucleus, unlike erythrocytes of the definitive cell line. Nucleated erythrocytes, interestingly, are normal throughout the life span of many nonmammalian genera, including reptiles, amphibians and birds. Definitive erythropoiesis is established in the liver and is characteristic of this and all subsequent sites of hematopoiesis. The morphologic maturation of this cell line, as it is found in adult marrow, is described in detail in Chapter 2 (see section 2.2.2). The relationship between primitive and definitive lineages, with respect to common or discrete precursor cells and the possibility that primitive cell line precursors may colonize sites of later definitive cell growth, has not been resolved.

1.4 Patterns of Hemoglobin Formation during Fetal and Early Neonatal Development

A striking biochemical characteristic of the hematopoietic cell system during fetal development in all mammals studied to date, including man, is conversion from the synthesis of embryonic hemoglobins to synthesis of adult hemoglobins (see section 8.2 for details of hemoglobin structure). In the human fetus, embryonic hemoglobins are first recognized between 4 and 6 weeks of gestation, at the time that the primitive cell lineage is established in the yolk sac (Fig. 1–2). From studies on the embryonic mouse, it now appears very likely that embryonic hemoglobins are produced by cells of the primitive lineage. These hemoglobins in man are called Gower I, a tetramer of four identical embryonic globin chains (ϵ_4), and Gower II, composed of two α chains and two ϵ chains ($\alpha_2\epsilon_2$) (Table 1–1). Later in fetal development, fetal hemoglobin (HbF), composed of two α chains and two γ chains ($\alpha_2\gamma_2$); adult hemoglobin (HbA; $\alpha_2\beta_2$); and the minor adult component HbA$_2$ ($\alpha_2\delta_2$) are synthesized. HbF is the major hemoglobin present at birth. Although called *fetal*, HbF is a normal adult hemoglobin, persisting as a minor component (less than 2–3%) throughout adult life. Synthesis of HbA may begin as early in fetal life as does that of HbF, i.e., by the 10th to 12th week of gestation. HbA does not, however, become the principal hemoglobin in circulating red blood cells until after birth. In normal adult blood, HbA accounts for about 95% of the hemoglobin. Under normal conditions this adult level is generally not reached until about 6 months after birth. Another minor component, HbA$_2$, normally accounts for less than 3% of hemoglobin in adult human subjects. From cytochemical studies it is known that both HbA and HbF are synthesized in the same cell. The proportions of HbA and HbF are not uniform from cell to cell in the normal adult.

Fig. 1–2.—Relative amounts of the several globin chains (ϵ, α, γ, β and δ) present during fetal development and the first year of life.

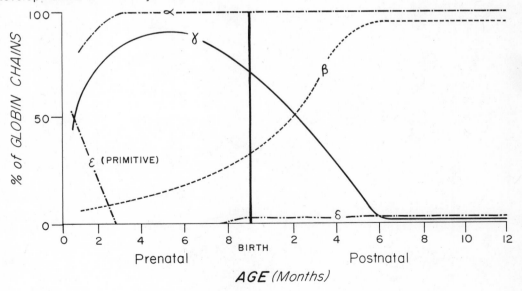

TABLE 1–1.—RELATIONSHIP
BETWEEN SITE OF ERYTHROPOIESIS
AND TYPE OF
HEMOGLOBIN FORMED

SITE OF ERYTHROPOIESIS	HEMOGLOBIN
Primitive (embryonic)	
Yolk sac blood islands	Gower I (ϵ_4)
	Gower II ($\alpha_2\epsilon_2$)
Definitive	
Liver (fetus)	Fetal ($\alpha_2\gamma_2$)
Spleen (fetus)	Adult ($\alpha_2\beta_2$)
Bone marrow (fetus and adult)	A_2 ($\alpha_2\delta_2$)

1.5 Regulation of Hematopoiesis

Erythrocytes, granulocytes and megakaryocytes develop from a common precursor or stem cell (Fig. 1–3). Evidence for a common precursor for the erythroid, myeloid and megakaryocytic cell lines derives from several types of experiments. Perhaps the most convincing is the observation that the hematopoietic tissues of lethally irradiated mice can be successfully "seeded" by injection of bone marrow cells from normal isogenic donors. These injected cells produce colo-

Fig. 1–3.—The sequential stages of maturation in hematopoiesis, emphasizing erythropoiesis. Stem cells are pluripotential. They differentiate into unipotential cells, which are the direct precursors of granulocytes (myeloblasts), platelets (megakaryoblasts) and red blood cells (RBC) (proerythroblasts). It is estimated that three to five cell divisions occur as proerythroblasts mature to the RBC stage. CFU = colony-forming units.

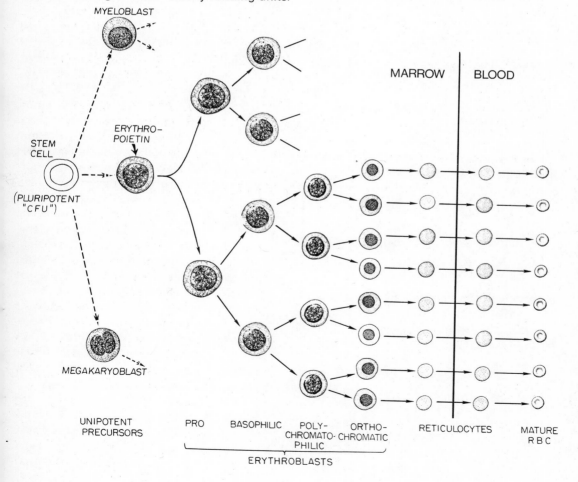

nies of hematopoietic cells in the spleen and marrow of the recipients. The individual colonies are of several types: pure erythroid, myeloid and megakaryocytic colonies or colonies containing mixed erythroid, myeloid and megakaryocytic cells. Chromosome markers introduced by x-irradiation of the donor cells provide clear-cut evidence that both the pure and the mixed colonies are, in fact, derived from a single donor stem cell.

These multipotential stem cells, sometimes referred to as colony-forming units (CFU), give rise to specialized precursor cells restricted to erythroid, myeloid or megakaryocytic differentiation (see Fig. 1–3). The rate of production of erythroid, myeloid and megakaryocytic cells from these specialized precursors appears to be determined in part by humoral substances. Substances acting selectively to stimulate erythropoiesis, granulopoiesis and thrombocytopoiesis have been described. They are referred to, respectively, as erythropoietin, granulopoietin and thrombopoietin. Of these hormonelike substances, erythropoietin is the most fully characterized. Indeed, at the present time the nature and physiologic role of granulopoietin and thrombopoietin are not established. We can consider the hormonal regulation of erythropoiesis as a potential paradigm for hematopoietic regulatory mechanisms.

1.5.1 REGULATION OF ERYTHROPOIESIS

Under normal conditions the circulating red cell mass is maintained within relatively narrow limits by adjustments in the rate of red cell production. It is generally agreed that the predominant control of erythropoiesis is mediated through alterations in tissue oxygen tension. A decrease in tissue oxygen tension, hypoxia, specifically in the kidney, is believed to lead to an increase in the activity of circulating erythropoietin. There are two major hypotheses with respect to the mechanism by which tissue hypoxia leads to an increase in the production of erythropoietin. On the one hand, hypoxia

may stimulate the kidney to secrete erythropoietin. On the other, the kidney may be stimulated to secrete an enzyme, erythrogenin, which is itself inactive in stimulating erythropoiesis but which reacts with a putative plasma substrate, erythropoietinogen, made in the liver and perhaps elsewhere as well, to produce active erythropoietin. There is insufficient evidence at present to permit a definitive decision between these two hypotheses.

1.5.2 CHARACTERIZATION OF ERYTHROPOIETIN

Erythropoietin can be measured by bioassay. The bioassay most commonly employed is one using as test animals mice whose endogenous erythropoiesis has been suppressed by polycythemia (which increases oxygen delivery). The stimulatory effect of erythropoietin on these animals is measured by determining the incorporation of ^{59}Fe into erythrocytes (see section 2.2.7.3). Assays have been developed that are sufficiently sensitive to detect normal levels of erythropoietin in both plasma and urine. Normal values of erythropoietin in men range between 1 and 4 units in a 24-hour urine sample. The level of erythropoietin in plasma and urine bears an inverse relationship to the hemoglobin level. However, in the presence of chronic hypoxemia due to residence at high altitude, chronic pulmonary insufficiency or right-to-left cardiovascular shunts, polycythemia (elevated red cell mass) may be associated with elevated erythropoietin levels. Certain tumors also are reported to be inappropriate producers of erythropoiesis-stimulating substances. Inappropriate low levels of erythropoietin are found in a wide variety of chronic inflammatory diseases and in advanced protein malnutrition.

Erythropoietin has not been completely purified. The hormone does appear to be relatively stable to heat. Chemically it is probably a glycoprotein containing sialic acid, hexosamine and possibly hexoses. The molecular weight has been variously estimated from as low as 25,000 to as high as 100,000. It migrates with α globulins on electrophoresis.

1.5.3 ACTION OF ERYTHROPOIETIN

The primary effect of erythropoietin appears to be to stimulate proliferation of the committed erythroid cell precursor. The hormone does not act directly to increase the rate of synthesis of globins. Rather, by increasing the proliferation of erythroid cell precursors, there is an increase in the number of cells capable of differentiating toward erythrocytes and synthesizing hemoglobin.

2

Erythroid Cell System: General Features and Introduction to the Problem of Anemia

2.1 Introduction

THE ERYTHROID CELL SYSTEM comprises the population of circulating red blood cells (RBC) and their nucleated precursors located in the normal adult in the bone marrow. A complex, and as yet not fully understood, homeostatic mechanism, involving in part the hormone, erythropoietin, operates upon the marrow precursors to maintain a circulating red cell population of a size and hemoglobin content adequate to preserve normal tissue oxygen tensions. The critical factor in the homeostatic mechanism regulating the production of erythropoietin is tissue oxygen tension, not red cell number or blood hemoglobin concentration (see section 1.5).

Anemia, defined as a lower than normal blood hemoglobin concentration (Hb) or packed red cell volume (hematocrit, Hct), occurs if red cell production is acutely or chronically insufficient to replace red cell losses — losses that may be due to normal red cell senescence, to accelerated red cell destruction (hemolysis) or to extracorporeal blood loss (bleeding). Some examples of anemia result from relatively uncomplicated alterations in single factors, e.g., the transient anemia following an acute hemorrhage in an otherwise healthy individual. In most

7

cases, however, the pathophysiology of anemia involves the interplay of several disturbances in red cell homeostasis, including limitations of production, as well as abnormal red cell survival. Our first obligation is to examine these factors in a general sense and to evaluate the significance and limitations of the technics at our disposal for distinguishing and quantitating them.

2.2 Red Cell Production

In the normal adult, red cell production is confined to the marrow of the axial skeleton and proximal long bones of the limbs. Under conditions of prolonged demand for accelerated erythropoiesis, the volume of active marrow may expand at the expense of normally fatty marrow and even, in growing children, at the expense of bony matrix. Under extreme and very prolonged stress, or in the face of marrow replacement by pathologic tissues, extramedullary sites such as spleen, lymph nodes and liver may develop foci of erythropoiesis. These extramedullary sites of hematopoiesis are the very organs responsible for blood cell production during embryonic life (see section 1.2). The erythropoietic tissues are capable of as much as a six- to eightfold increase in red cell production in response to the stimulus of anemia. Indeed, even under conditions of accelerated blood destruction, blood hemoglobin concentration may remain at near normal levels as long as the rate of destruction does not exceed the capacity for compensatory expansion of the red cell precursor population.

2.2.1 EFFECTS OF ERYTHROPOIETIN

As already noted, the mass of the erythropoietic tissue appears to be physiologically under the control of the hormone erythropoietin, whose production is intimately related to the tissue oxygen tension (see section 1.5.1). Although the mechanism of action of the hormone is by no means fully understood, one major effect appears to be upon the proliferation of early erythroid precursor cells. Differentiation of these precursors by an orderly and recognizable series of sequential stages of functional specialization, characterized by both morphologic and biochemical features, is part of the response of the hematopoietic tissues to the hormone.

The process of erythropoietic differentiation can be traced from the common hematopoietic stem cell. This cell is recognized only by its functional properties (see Chapter 1); morphologic identification has not been achieved. The stem cell is capable of differentiating along the erythroid, granulocytic or megakaryocytic pathways, but the signals or triggers that define which pathway is chosen by a given stem cell have not been established. The earliest identifiable committed erythropoietic precursor is a cell that, in the presence of erythropoietin, can proliferate and form clones of erythroid cells.

2.2.2 MORPHOLOGY OF ERYTHROPOIESIS

The first morphologically recognized erythroid element is the *proerythroblast* (Fig. 2–1, A). Maturation of the proerythroblast to the circulating red cell involves four or five cell divisions (see Fig. 1–3); production of characteristic red cell proteins (hemoglobin and enzymes), surface antigens and metabolic machinery; loss of replicative capacity and eventually of the nucleus itself; and acquisition of characteristic red cell morphology. The process takes between 48 and 96 hours and one proerythroblast will give rise to 16–32 progeny erythrocytes. The proerythroblast is a large cell (mean diameter 25μ) displaying a high nucleo-cytoplasmic ratio; the nucleus contains predominantly extended chromatin and contains one or more large nucleoli. DNA, RNA and protein synthesis are active, but hemoglobin synthesis is not detected.

The proerythroblast stage is succeeded by the *basophilic erythroblast* (see Fig. 2–1, B). The basophilic erythroblast is basophilic

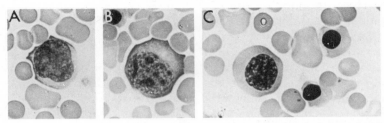

Fig. 2–1.—Sequence of maturation of erythroid precursor cells during normal erythropoiesis. **A,** proerythroblast; **B,** basophilic erythroblast; **C,** polychromatic erythroblast *(left)* and two orthochromatic erythroblasts *(right)*.

Fig. 2–2.—Appearance of normal red blood cells and red cells displaying a variety of morphologic stigmata seen in hematologic disorders. **A,** normal red blood cells; **B,** moderate anisocytosis and poikilocytosis; **C,** microspherocytes; **D,** hypochromic leptocytes in β-thalassemia; **E,** hypochromia with anisocytosis, microcytosis and elliptocytes in iron deficiency; **F,** macroovalocytes in megaloblastic anemia; **G,** fragmented schistocytes; **H,** target cells; **I,** two irreversibly sickled red cells and a nucleated red cell in sickle cell disease; **J,** tear-drop red cell.

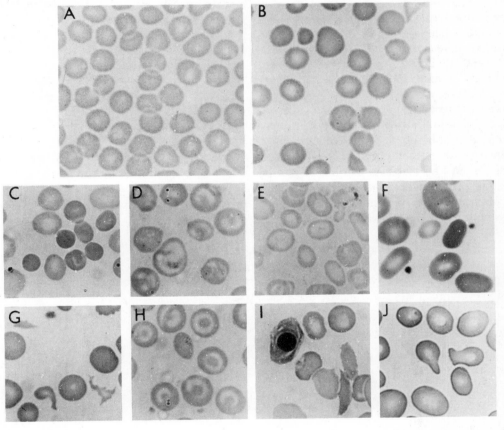

because of the high concentration of cytoplasmic ribosomes that accumulate in preparation for the onset of hemoglobin synthesis, which marks the *polychromatophilic erythroblast* stage (see Fig. 2–1, C) of development. These cells display increasingly deep staining for hemoglobin (acidophilia by the Wright stain or a positive reaction with the benzidine reagent) and a progressive decrease in the concentration of cytoplasmic ribosomes. With maturation, the nucleus becomes increasingly pyknotic. Cell division continues until the *orthochromatic erythroblast* stage (see Fig. 2–1, C), by which time the cytoplasm has lost much of its basophilia, although hemoglobin synthesis continues on relatively stable ribosome-globin messenger RNA (mRNA) complexes. At this stage the nucleus is expelled and the nuclear remnant is phagocytosed by macrophages. The cytoplasmic moiety forms the *reticulocyte* (see section 2.2.7.1). This non-nucleated cell still contains active hemoglobin-synthesizing polyribosomes as well as mitochondria. At this stage the reticulocytes are released into the circulation. During the first 24–36 hours of circulation in the blood, the reticulocyte is transformed into the mature erythrocyte (Fig. 2–2). This transformation is characterized by progressive decrease in the number of polyribosomes and mitochondria and by loss of hemoglobin synthetic capacity.

2.2.3 Synthesis of Macromolecules during Erythroid Cell Differentiation

As erythroid cells differentiate from the immature precursor to mature, non-nucleated RBC, there are sequential changes in a number of metabolic and biosynthetic capabilities (Table 2–1). These biochemical events are accompanied by the morphologic changes characteristic of erythroid differentiation, but it is not possible precisely to correlate the biochemical and morphologic changes. Proerythroblasts, basophilic erythroblasts and polychromatophilic erythroblasts, as already noted, have the capacity for *cell division* but there is a progressive decrease in the rate of DNA synthesis. The orthochromatic erythroblast has lost the capacity for DNA synthesis and mitosis. *RNA,* including ribosomal (rRNA), transfer (tRNA) and mRNA, is produced through the late polychromatophilic and perhaps into the early orthochromatic erythroblast stage. The reticulocyte has no nucleus and does not synthesize RNA. mRNA for globin, the protein moiety of hemoglobin, is first synthesized in basophilic erythroblasts and accumulates through the orthochromatic erythroblast stage.

Globin synthesis begins in the basophilic erythroblasts and continues until the reticu-

TABLE 2–1.—METABOLIC CHANGES ASSOCIATED WITH
ERYTHROID CELL DIFFERENTIATION*

STAGE	PROERYTH-ROBLAST	BASOPHILIC ERYTHROBLAST	POLYCHROMATOPHILIC ERYTHROBLAST	ORTHOCHROMATIC ERYTHROBLAST	RETICU-LOCYTE	YOUNG RBC
DNA Synthesis	+ +	+	+	0	0	0
rRNA† and tRNA† synthesis	+ +	+	+	0	0	0
Globin mRNA† synthesis	±	+ +	+	+	0	0
Heme synthesis	+ +	+ +	+	+	0	0
Oxidative phosphorylation	+ +	+ +	+ +	+	±	0
Cytochrome system	+ +	+ +	+ +	+ +	+	0
Lipid synthesis	+ +	+ +	+ +	+ +	+	0
Tricarboxylic acid cycle	+ +	+ +	+ +	+ +	+	0
Anaerobic glycolysis	+ +	+ +	+ +	+ +	+	0
Pentose phosphate pathway	+ +	+ +	+ +	+ +	+ +	+

*Relative metabolic activities are designated on a scale of 0 (no activity) to + + (fully active).
†rRNA = ribosomal RNA; tRNA = transfer RNA; mRNA = messenger RNA.

locyte matures to the erythrocyte. It is estimated that as much as 15–20% of the total hemoglobin in mature erythrocytes is formed during the reticulocyte stage. Globin production constitutes a very large fraction (about 95%) of the protein synthesis in maturing erythroid cells. A number of possible molecular mechanisms could account for the predominant synthesis of one class of protein. A crucial question is the number of copies of the globin genes in the genome. There are fewer than 20, and possibly fewer than 10, structural genes for globins in the haploid human chromosome, and there is no evidence that the number changes during differentiation. It appears that the large amount of globin synthesized during erythroid cell differentiation reflects selective rates of transcription, processing or translation of globin mRNA, and not gene amplification or gene reiteration.

2.2.4 GLOBIN MESSENGER RNA

Globin mRNA, purified from human or other animal erythroid cells, can be added to an in vitro cell-free system for protein synthesis and will direct the formation of complete globin chains. Globin mRNA has been partially characterized chemically and physically. It has a molecular weight of approximately 200,000 daltons. Since human globin chains contain from 143–146 amino acids, assuming that each amino acid is coded by three nucleotide bases, each with an average molecular weight of 300, the molecular weight of mRNA coding for a single globin chain should be only 125,000–130,000 daltons ($300 \times 3 \times 143$–146). The nature and function of that portion of globin mRNA apparently in excess of that required to code for the amino acid sequence of globin are unknown. There is evidence that a portion of this "excess" mRNA consists of adenylic acid sequences, and there is speculation that polyadenylate sequences may be important in determining the life span of mRNA. mRNA for globin, as are other eukaryotic

mRNA for specialized proteins, is relatively long lived. This is supported, for example, by the fact that reticulocytes, which synthesize no RNA, continue to synthesize globin.

2.2.5 GLOBIN SYNTHESIS

In normal erythroid cells the rates of synthesis of the two principal globins, called α and β, are very close to equal. In the adult the rates of synthesis of δ and γ chains (which are part of the two minor adult hemoglobins, $A_2[\alpha_2\delta_2]$ and $F[\alpha_2\gamma_2]$; see section 8.2) are considerably lower than α or β globin synthesis. There is evidence that this is due to a smaller amount of mRNA for δ globin and γ globin in the adult erythroblast, compared with mRNA for α and β globin. There are genetic diseases of globin chain synthesis (the thalassemias; see section 8.7) that are characterized by pathologically decreased amounts of mRNA for specific globin chains.

2.2.6 HEME SYNTHESIS

The hemoglobin molecule contains four heme groups, one bound to each of the four globin chains of hemoglobin (see section 8.2 and Figs. 8–2 and 8–3). Heme is also a prosthetic group for proteins other than hemoglobin (including myoglobin) enzymes, such as catalase and peroxidase, and cytochromes.

Heme is composed of four pyrrole rings, coordinated through their substituent nitrogen atoms to an iron (see Fig. 8–2). The pyrrole molecule itself has a sequence of alternating single and double bonds; the conjugated double bonds are responsible for absorption of visible light and for the red color of hemoglobin. The absorption spectrum of oxyhemoglobin has two maxima in the visible region, one between 540 nm and 576 nm, the other between 412 nm and 415 nm. The former is due to the metalloporphyrin, the latter to the conjugated ring structure of the pyrrole portion of the molecule.

The biosynthesis of heme involves a number of steps, each catalyzed by a separate enzyme (Fig. 2–3). Succinyl coenzyme A and glycine, formed in the tricarboxylic acid cycle, are condensed to form Δ-aminolevulinic acid (ALA). There is evidence that the enzyme catalyzing this reaction, ALA synthetase, is rate limiting in the pathway of heme synthesis. Pyridoxal phosphate is a coenzyme at this step in heme synthesis. It is of interest that some anemias have been reported to respond to administration of the vitamin, pyridoxine or pyridoxal phosphate (see section 4.4.3). Two ALA molecules condense to form porphobilinogen. In turn, four molecules of porphobilinogen condense to form the tetrapyrrole, uroporphyrinogen. Uroporphyrinogen is decarboxylated and

converted to coproporphyrinogen and, in turn, to protoporphyrin. The final step in the heme synthetic pathway is the insertion of ferrous iron into protoporphyrin, catalyzed by the enzyme, ferrochelatase. The formation of ALA and conversion of coproporphyrinogen to protoporphyrin and heme take place in the mitochondria.

2.2.7 PARAMETERS OF RED CELL PRODUCTION

2.2.7.1 RETICULOCYTE COUNT.—This is the most commonly used method for evaluating the marrow's response to anemic stress. Reticulocytes are stained by a supravital technic that depends on the precipitation of dye with reticulocyte ribosomes. Reticulo-

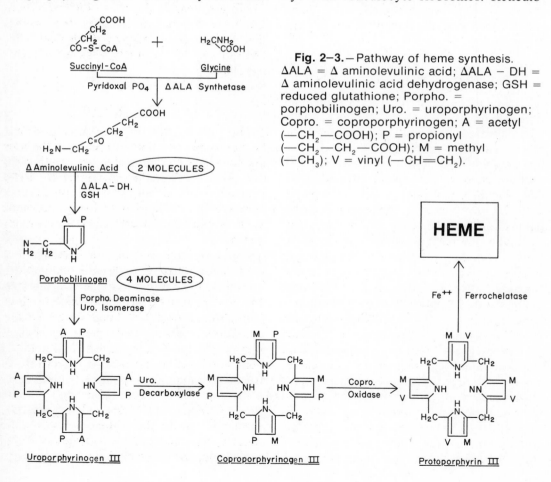

Fig. 2–3.—Pathway of heme synthesis. ΔALA = Δ aminolevulinic acid; ΔALA − DH = Δ aminolevulinic acid dehydrogenase; GSH = reduced glutathione; Porpho. = porphobilinogen; Uro. = uroporphyrinogen; Copro. = coproporphyrinogen; A = acetyl ($-CH_2-COOH$); P = propionyl ($-CH_2-CH_2-COOH$); M = methyl ($-CH_3$); V = vinyl ($-CH=CH_2$).

cytes are counted and expressed as a percentage of the mature RBC. The normal reticulocyte count is about 1%. Reticulocytes mature to erythrocytes in $1 - 1\frac{1}{2}$ days (or somewhat longer if the reticulocytes are released prematurely under the stress of severe anemia and high titers of erythropoietin).

Under the conditions of accelerated red cell production, reticulocytes constitute a higher than normal percentage of the red cell population, if the products of erythroid cell maturation are being effectively delivered to the peripheral blood. In using the reticulocyte count as a reflection of marrow erythropoiesis, it is essential to take into consideration the level of the Hct or RBC count. Since reticulocytes are expressed as a percentage of total red cells, the reticulocyte count may be overestimated in the presence of severe anemia (reduced number of mature red cells). The reticulocyte count (%) may be "corrected" for anemia as follows:

ulocytic white blood cells [WBC]; see section 9.2) in the normal marrow is approximately 1:3. Granulocyte precursors are more numerous than erythroid precursors in the marrow, even though there are fewer of them in the circulating blood. The life span of granulocytes is much shorter and their turnover rate much higher. Changes in the E:G ratio may reflect alterations in either the erythroid or granulocytic compartments of the marrow, or both. The ratio rarely can provide more than inferential evidence as to the absolute size of either compartment. Nevertheless, a marrow examination that indicates a relative increase in erythroid elements *(erythroid hyperplasia)*, in the presence of anemia and in the absence of evidence for suppression of granulopoiesis, is strong evidence for accelerated erythropoiesis. Quantitation is crude at best, and interpretation may be difficult in the face of other complicating hematopoietic abnormalities. Of par-

$$\text{Corrected count (\%)} = \text{observed count (\%)} \times \frac{\text{patient's Hct}}{\text{normal Hct}}$$

The presence of large red cells (macrocytes) displaying polychromasia (bluish tint) in the circulation is suggestive of the accelerated release of immature RBC from the marrow. These cells are not necessarily all reticulocytes, but their presence suggests elevated erythropoietin activity and should prompt performance of a reticulocyte count.

Mild elevation of the reticulocyte count also may be the consequence of infiltration of the marrow by tumor, fibrosis or granuloma, with or without extramedullary hematopoiesis. Under these circumstances there also may be nucleated red cells and immature white cell precursors in the circulation, and red cell morphology usually is abnormal (teardrop shapes).

2.2.7.2 ERYTHROID:GRANULOCYTIC (E:G) RATIO OF BONE MARROW. — The ratio of nucleated red cell precursors to granulocytic elements (the precursors of circulating gran-

ticular significance, however, is erythroid hyperplasia in the marrow accompanied by a low reticulocyte count in the peripheral blood. This observation provides the clinical evidence for *ineffective erythropoiesis*. In normal marrow at least 80 – 90% of developing erythroblasts produce circulating reticulocytes and red cells. Under certain pathologic conditions, e.g., pernicious anemia and thalassemia, vigorous marrow erythropoietic activity is accompanied by considerable intra-marrow erythroid cell destruction and failure of reticulocyte release, which is what is meant by the term ineffective erythropoiesis.

2.2.7.3 FERROKINETIC STUDIES. — Iron is a prerequisite for synthesis of the heme moiety of hemoglobin, and the kinetics of iron metabolism may be useful in assessing red cell production. To evaluate iron metabolism, a tracer dose of ^{59}Fe, bound to human plasma transferrin (the iron-binding and -transporting protein of plasma), is injected into the circulation. Repeated samples are withdrawn and the clearance rate of plasma iron (half-time [$t^{1/2}$] of disappearance of radioactivity) determined. Accelerated clearance rates (shortened $t^{1/2}$) are almost always the consequence of accelerated erythropoiesis, whether effective or ineffective. The $t^{1/2}$ ^{59}Fe, in conjunction with the level of plasma iron, may be transformed mathematically into an index of plasma iron turnover (mg of iron/100 ml blood/day). The reutilization of tracer iron released from red cells as they reach the end of their life span (see section 2.3) makes this test rather less valuable clinically than might be predicted.

Determination of ^{59}Fe in samples of RBC withdrawn at intervals over the 4–10 days after administration of a tracer dose of the isotope provides an estimate of iron utilization by erythroid cells and may be interpreted as a measure of *effective erythropoiesis* (i.e., erythropoiesis that results in viable, circulating RBC). In normal persons, red cell ^{59}Fe radioactivity rises steadily from about 24 hours after administration of the tracer, and the percentage utilization of the administered dose reaches a maximum (about 80%) between the 10th and 14th days. Rapid iron clearance (high plasma iron turnover), accompanied by rapid and high iron utilization, indicates accelerated effective erythropoiesis. Ineffective erythropoiesis is characterized by rapid iron clearance associated with reduced and delayed iron utilization. Interpretation of iron kinetics data is particularly difficult in the presence of rapid peripheral red cell destruction (accelerated hemolysis), since labeled iron, removed from the hemolyzed blood by the reticuloendothelial system, is reutilized by the erythropoietic tissues. In the presence of active bleeding from any source, interpretation of iron kinetics is not valid.

^{59}Fe is a gamma-emitter and, by means of well-collimated scanners, the distribution of ^{59}Fe in various organs can be estimated by body surface counting. This technic may provide information of value in assessing extramedullary sites of erythropoiesis, e.g., in cases of myeloid metaplasia and aplastic anemia.

2.3 Red Cell Life Span and Destruction

The normal erythrocyte circulates in the blood stream with a life span of 100–120 days, at which time the senescent red cells are selectively sequestered and destroyed by the reticuloendothelial system of macrophages. The spleen plays the predominant role in the destruction of normally senescent red cells, although other reticuloendothelial organs, notably the liver, are competent to assume this responsibility following splenectomy. The signal that indicates that a given red cell is senescent and ready for phagocytosis is not understood. A variety of changes in red cell enzymes occurs during its circulating life span, and some of these are likely to be of critical importance in maintaining normal red cell integrity (see Table 2–1). Factors that may be significant in this regard are oxidation-reduction systems that maintain hemoglobin in the reduced (ferrous iron) state (see section 7.1); energy sources critical for ion transfer across the cell membrane and for maintenance of the appropriate ionic and osmotic gradients (see section 7.1); and enzymes that may be implicated in preserving normal red cell plasma membrane composition and physical properties. Although no single factor has yet been identified that is the sine qua non of red cell senescence, it has been clearly demonstrated that red cells undergo progressive changes in their physical properties, including loss of pliability, decrease in surface charge and probably an increase in methemoglobin (ferric hemoglobin) content, as they reach the end of their normal life span. Details of some of these features of red cell metabolism and aging will be covered in subsequent sections (see Chapter 7). The best interpretation of available data suggests that all or many of these changes may contribute to progressive inability of the red cell to flow rapidly through the splenic pulp. Red cells that have lost flexibility and have decreased surface charge, and perhaps other still unrecognized defects, are retarded in their passage through the splenic red pulp, particularly through the reticulum-laced interstices of the Billroth cords. The environment of the splenic pulp, principally low glucose concentration, mild hypoxia, hypercapnia and relatively low pH, is deleterious to red cells. At some critical stage of aging, these conditions accelerate the deterioration of red cell homeostasis and render the cell liable to phagocytosis by one of the numerous splenic macrophages.

Within the macrophage, ingested red cells are subject to proteolytic and lipolytic enzymes. Much of the iron released from heme is reutilized for synthesis of new hemoglobin in the marrow. The porphyrin moiety of heme (pyrrole pigment) is not reutilized. The porphyrin ring is broken and reduced to bilirubin. Released bilirubin is bound to serum albumin, transported to and conjugated by the liver and excreted as the gluconate into the bile. About 6 gm of hemoglobin is normally catabolized daily, producing some 200 mg of bilirubin. The normal serum level of unconjugated bilirubin in transit to the liver does not exceed about 0.6 mg/100 ml. Conjugated bilirubin in the intestinal lumen is metabolized to urobilinogen by bacteria; a fraction of this is reabsorbed and reexcreted, in part by the liver and filtered in part into the urine.

Accelerated red cell destruction, by increasing the load of bilirubin for hepatic clearance, frequently leads to elevation of the serum level of unconjugated bilirubin and increased urinary excretion of urobilinogen. A chronically elevated bilirubin excretion rate may result in precipitation of bilirubin stones in the gallbladder and the symptoms of cholelithiasis.

A wide variety of injuries and metabolic defects may result in premature red cell destruction, i.e., *hemolytic anemia*. The nature of these specific injuries is the subject of Chapters 6–8. Nevertheless certain generalizations can be made that help synthesize an approach to clinical evaluation of hemolytic anemia. In general, red cell injuries, whether a consequence of inherited defects or acquired lesions, result in erythrocytes that are abnormal with respect to shape, rigidity or surface properties, any one or all of which predispose to premature entrapment by the reticuloendothelial system. In general, relatively mild injuries result in an acceleration of splenic sequestration and erythrophagocytosis. More severe injury results in erythrophagocytosis by other portions of the reticuloendothelial system, particularly the liver, which because of its size and blood flow can be a major and at times the predominant organ of erythrophagocytosis. It is this capacity for activation of the hepatic reticuloendothelial system that sometimes obviates the effect of a splenectomy performed to alleviate hemolytic anemia. Accelerated hemolysis that is mediated principally by erythrophagocytosis is commonly called *extravascular hemolysis*.

Intravascular hemolysis refers to the lysis of erythrocytes while in the circulation, with consequent release of red cell contents directly into the plasma. Intravascular hemolysis is rarely a major component of hemolytic anemia, but may occur, for example, following transfusion with a major blood group incompatibility, following burns or during severe Plasmodium infection. *Paroxysmal nocturnal hemoglobinuria* is another unusual intravascular hemolytic condition of complex pathophysiology and protean hematologic manifestations (see section 6.8). The red cells in this disorder have an acquired sensitivity to hemolytic complement.

Hemoglobin released during intravascular hemolysis is promptly bound to the plasma protein, haptoglobin; the hemoglobin-haptoglobin complex is cleared from the blood by the reticuloendothelial system, and the plasma haptoglobin level is sharply reduced. There is a limit to the haptoglobin-hemoglobin-binding capacity (normally 150 mg hemoglobin/100 ml of plasma), and hemoglobin released in excess of this is handled in a different fashion. Some is degraded in the circulation, and the heme moiety, as hematin, combines with albumin to form methemalbumin. Free hemoglobin also is filtered by the glomerulus; of this, a portion reaches the voided urine as hemoglobin and methemoglobin, whereas some is reabsorbed and degraded by renal tubular cells. These tubular cells accumulate hemosiderin; desquamated tubular cells containing hemosiderin may be passed into the urine *(hemosiderinuria).*

Although severe intravascular hemolysis is rare, mild degrees of intravascular hemolysis, sufficient to depress the normal plasma haptoglobin level and even to produce minor degrees of hemosiderinuria, accompany many instances of extravascular hemolysis.

Recognition of a state of accelerated hemolysis, and assessment of its severity, is an essential part of the evaluation of any anemia. The results of such studies may have the most profound therapeutic implications. Both direct and indirect parameters are useful in demonstrating and documenting accelerated hemolysis.

2.3.1 DIRECT EVIDENCE FOR ACCELERATED HEMOLYSIS

2.3.1.1 RED CELL LIFE SPAN STUDIES.— Two basic approaches to the determination of red cell life span have been employed, but only the ^{51}Cr technic is now used clinically.

2.3.1.1.1 Cohort-labeling.— When a short pulse of labeled glycine (^{14}C- or ^{15}N-glycine) is administered, the label is incorporated into erythroblasts synthesizing hemoglobin and retained by the progeny erythrocytes until they are destroyed. By this means it is possible to determine the life span of a cohort of cells, all of them labeled at the very beginning of their development. Isotope determinations (by radioactivity or mass spectroscopy) on samples of circulating blood provide

the characteristic normal curve of red cell survival illustrated in Fig. 2–4, A. ^{59}Fe is not a useful label for life span studies because of the reutilization of iron (see section 2.2.7.3).

In the presence of accelerated hemolysis, two patterns may be found (Fig. 2–4, B). As indicated by the solid line, the life span may be shortened by virtue of a uniform, age-dependent, premature senescence of all red cells of the labeled cohort. Although this hypothetical pattern is rarely perfectly duplicated in clinical situations, the shortened life span observed in the hereditary hemolytic anemia due to glucose 6-phosphate dehydrogenase (G-6-PD) deficiency may approach this mode. The dashed line in Figure 2–4, B, alternatively, represents the survival curve when hemolysis occurs by the random destruction of red cells, independent of their age. Antibody-mediated hemolytic anemias and hemolysis secondary to some of the abnormal hemoglobins exemplify this pattern of hemolysis to some extent. In clinical practice cohort labeling, although extremely informative, is not used; radioactive ^{14}C is not justifiably administered to otherwise healthy individuals (due to its long half-life and widespread distribution in tissues), and

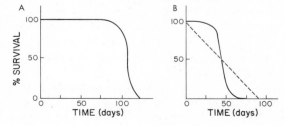

Fig. **2–4.**—*A,* normal red cell life span, determined by the disappearance from the circulation of radioactive glycine, incorporated into red cell hemoglobin on day zero. Sudden disappearance of labeled hemoglobin between days 100 and 120 reflects the destruction of a cohort of normally senescent red cells. *B,* shortened red cell life span (accelerated hemolysis) determined by the cohort labeling technic. Red cell age-dependent hemolysis *(solid line)* and random hemolysis *(dashed line)* show different isotope-disappearance curves.

^{15}N and mass spectroscopy is prohibitively expensive.

2.3.1.1.2 Labeling of mixed-age populations. — Labeling of an age-randomized population of red cells in the peripheral blood may readily be achieved by incubation of an aliquot of patient's blood with isotopic sodium chromate (^{51}Cr). Chromate is bound to hemoglobin. Labeled cells are reinfused and their fate ascertained by periodic assay of the radioactivity of sampled blood. Since red cells of all ages are randomly labeled, the theoretical radioactivity-disappearance curve has the shape indicated in Figure 2–5 (solid curve). A half-disappearance time of 60 days would be anticipated for normal blood. However, ^{51}Cr is eluted from circulating red cells at a rate of about 1% per day; this elution results in an observed disappearance curve (dashed line) such that the normal ^{51}Cr half-disappearance time is only 28–32 days.

Although ^{51}Cr labeling has some drawbacks and does not provide an absolute measure of true life span, it has proved the single

Fig. 2–5. — Red cell life span as determined by the disappearance of ^{51}Cr from the circulation. Labeled chromate is bound to the hemoglobin of all red cells in an aliquot, independent of red cell age. Radioactivity disappears from the circulation as a function of both hemolysis and elution of ^{51}Cr, hence the difference between the theoretical *(solid line)* and observed *(dashed line)* curves of isotope disappearance.

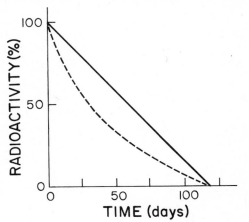

most precise method for detecting a shortened red cell survival time in clinical situations. The t$^{1/2}$ ^{51}Cr is not accurate in the face of acutely changing rates of hemolysis (nonsteady state) and is uninterpretable in the presence of bleeding. The value of the ^{51}Cr technic may be extended by means of surface counting to provide an estimation of the relative contributions of the spleen and liver to red cell sequestration. This information may be of prognostic value in considering splenectomy for alleviation of hemolysis.

2.3.2 INDIRECT INDICATIONS OF ACCELERATED HEMOLYSIS

The measurement of t$^{1/2}$ ^{51}Cr is the most direct clinical evidence for shortened red cell life span, but it is not routinely necessary to perform this test simply to determine whether accelerated hemolysis is present. A constellation of more indirect but simpler tests may provide completely satisfactory, albeit inferential, evidence for a hemolytic state.

2.3.2.1 MEASUREMENTS OF THE CATABOLIC PRODUCTS OF HEMOLYSIS. — *2.3.2.1.1 Serum unconjugated bilirubin and bilirubin metabolites.* — The normal unconjugated bilirubin level is about 0.5 mg/100 ml serum. In the presence of accelerated hemolysis, the serum unconjugated bilirubin may range from near normal levels to as much as 3.5–4 mg/100 ml, the level depending in large part upon hepatic conjugating capacity and rate of hemolysis. Higher levels of unconjugated bilirubin raise the possibility of concomitant liver disease. Elevated unconjugated bilirubin levels may result either from hemolysis (extravascular or intravascular) or from ineffective erythropoiesis.

Bilirubin, conjugated by the liver and secreted into the gut, is converted to fecal urobilinogen. This product also may be measured. Elevated levels indicate an acceleration of porphyrin pigment metabolism, probably due to accelerated hemolysis. Reabsorbed urobilinogen may be excreted into the urine, and an elevated urine urobilinogen level has the same implication.

2.3.2.1.2 Estimation of serum haptoglobin. — This test in principle depends upon the hemoglobin-binding capacity of the protein and upon the electrophoretic determination of bound and free hemoglobin. The serum sample is mixed with hemoglobin to form the hemoglobin-haptoglobin complex. The complex moves as an α_2 globulin and the haptoglobin level is determined as the amount of benzidine-reactive protein migrating with the α_2 globulins. Free hemoglobin migrates in the β globulin region; full saturation of haptoglobin is signaled by the appearance of stainable free hemoglobin on the electrophorogram. The concentration of haptoglobin is expressed as milligrams of hemoglobin-binding capacity/100 ml of serum. Other methods of determination of haptoglobin levels are also available. Occasionally, reduced haptoglobin levels have been noted in hepatocellular disease, and congenital absence of the protein is described. Increased haptoglobin is observed during infections, inflammatory disorders, malignancies and probably other conditions. A normal haptoglobin level in the face of evidence for hemolysis may be due to such complicating conditions, which elevate the haptoglobin concentration.

2.3.2.1.3 Estimation of plasma hemoglobin. — This test depends on the catalytic action of heme proteins on the oxidation of benzidine by hydrogen peroxide, a reaction measured by the intensity of the blue-to-violet color of oxidized benzidine. Avoiding accidental hemolysis of the blood sample during the preparation of plasma is critical. A significantly elevated level of plasma hemoglobin denotes intravascular hemolysis.

2.3.2.1.4 Methemalbuminemia. — This is determined spectroscopically (absorption band at 558 nm of the ammonium hemochromogen derivative; so-called Schumm's test) and is observed in the presence of intravascular hemolysis following saturation and depletion of plasma haptoglobin.

2.3.2.1.5 Hemosiderinuria. — Hemosiderin in the urinary sediment is recognized by staining a smear of sediment with the Prussian blue reagent and searching for blue granules. It is particularly useful in detecting chronic but intermittent intravascular hemolysis since the test may be positive even after hemolysis has stopped.

2.3.2.2 TESTS REFLECTING AN ACCELERATED RATE OF ERYTHROPOIESIS. — *2.3.2.2.1 Reticulocyte count.* — It should be recalled that the corrected level of circulating reticulocytes is a parameter of red cell production rate (see section 2.2.7.1). An elevated reticulocyte count (and the presence of polychromasia) often is adduced as evidence for hemolytic anemia. It should be borne in mind that this is an inferential conclusion; an elevated red cell production rate is an indicator of accelerated hemolysis only if (1) there is no bleeding, and (2) the increased production is not the result of repair of a prior block to normal red cell maturation. Reticulocytosis will follow replacement of iron, vitamin B_{12} or folic acid in a patient depleted of one of these nutrients, for example. At times, simply the institution of an adequate hospital diet in a malnourished patient may trigger a reticulocyte response that can be misinterpreted as a sign of hemolysis unless good judgment is exercised. It should be remembered also that a "normal" reticulocyte count in the presence of anemia is abnormal since the marrow *should* respond by an accelerated production of reticulocytes.

2.3.2.2.2 Nucleated red blood cells (NRBC). — NRBC also may be released prematurely (i.e., before their enucleation) under conditions of prolonged and severe hemolytic stress. Under these circumstances the reticulocyte count also is quite elevated. On the other hand, in some situations NRBC are found in the peripheral blood in the presence of only a minimally elevated reticulocyte count. This occurs with *extramedullary erythropoiesis,* i.e., erythropoiesis outside the marrow (e.g., in spleen, liver and lymph nodes). The regulation of release of blood cells in these extramedullary sites is imperfect, and immature forms escape into the blood. In addition to NRBC, immature granulocytes and large immature platelets often are seen in the blood in this situation. Extramedullary hematopoiesis is prominent when the marrow is infiltrated with abnormal tissues, which may be neoplastic (metastatic carcinoma, lymphoma), granulomatous (tuberculosis, sarcoidosis) or fibrotic (myelofibrosis with myeloid metaplasia). NRBC also are commonly found in the peripheral blood in severe examples of ineffective erythropoiesis.

2.3.2.2.3 Erythroid hyperplasia of the bone marrow. — See section 2.2.7.2.

2.4 General Approach to the Evaluation of Anemia

Anemia, meaning a *lower than normal* circulating red cell mass, is by definition a clinical sign, not a diagnostic entity. The routine clinical parameters used in assaying for anemia are the hemoglobin concentrations (gm of Hb/100 ml of whole blood), Hct (volume of packed red cells/volume of whole blood, expressed as a percentage) and RBC count (number of RBC/cu mm of whole blood). Criteria of "normality" vary, depending upon many local conditions, but for practical purposes in most U. S. communities, normal values are as given in the Appendix. At birth these values are somewhat higher, as is the reticulocyte count. During the pediatric ages the normal levels are somewhat lower, approaching adult levels after puberty (see Appendix). These figures provide guidelines only. As in so many aspects of medicine, the most useful value for normal may be the patient's own level at a prior time of good health. Deviations from this are potentially of far greater use to the physician than are deviations from an arbitrary norm.

Is there "significant" anemia? In asking this critical question, we are really asking two independent questions and both must be

answered before either dismissing a laboratory value as insignificant or embarking upon a diagnostic evaluation. The components of this question are in reality:

1. *Is the anemia of significant magnitude to be a factor contributing to the patient's symptoms or to the progress of illness?*

The answer to this question will be found in part by considering the absolute magnitude and rate of development of the anemia; the nature of the basic disease; the contribution of tissue hypoxia to its pathophysiology and the cardiovascular, renal and cerebral circulatory status of the patient. In general, mild degrees of anemia (Hb 10 – 14 gm/100 ml) are usually asymptomatic except in the presence of heavy effort or impaired cardiovascular or respiratory function. Quite surprising degrees of anemia can be tolerated, at least at rest, in the presence of good cardiovascular reserve, if the anemia is developed gradually. Cardiovascular adjustments, including increased cardiac output and vascular shunting, do not fully account for the ability to sustain tolerable oxygenation despite anemia. The paradox is at least partially resolved by the fact that hemoglobin decreases its oxygen affinity in the presence of hypoxia from any cause. This property, the ability to alter the position of the oxygen dissociation curve, is the consequence of reversible binding of organic phosphates, principally 2,3-diphosphoglycerate, to deoxyhemoglobin. This will be discussed further (see section 8.2.1).

2. *Is the anemia "significant," whatever its magnitude, in that it directs our attention to an underlying pathologic process?*

The anemia itself may be "insignificant" in the sense of question 1 and yet be a major diagnostic clue to the existence and nature of either hematologic or nonhematologic disease.

Determination of the particular mechanism(s) and specific etiology of an anemia requires the logical and considered use of a variety of laboratory procedures in conjunction with a careful history and physical examination. By strictly adhering to the injunction, first, to establish the pathophysiologic mechanism of the anemia (i.e., blood loss, decreased production, disordered maturation or accelerated hemolysis) and then to determine the specific etiologic factors or lesions, it is possible to work up an anemia with an efficiency rarely matched in clinical practice. One example of an anemia "flowsheet," based upon principal pathophysiologic mechanisms, is illustrated in Table 2–2. Since many anemias are the result of complicated pathophysiologic mechanisms, this classification must be treated only as a first approximation.

2.5 Clinical History

Anemia may be suspected because of symptoms (e.g., weakness, fatigue, dyspnea), physical findings of pallor and tissue anoxia or it may be discovered fortuitously during a screening laboratory examination. A summary of some of the protean manifestations of this frequent clinical problem is provided in Table 2–3.

A proper clinical evaluation of anemia cannot be confined to these relatively direct manifestations of the anemia itself. The patient's history also must be searched to elicit features that will help unravel the not infrequently complex pathophysiology of anemia. The perceptiveness of the history and physical examination will depend in large part upon familiarity with the disease patterns and pathogenic mechanisms associated with specific anemias, such as those treated in greater detail later in this text.

Several points may be advanced, however, in a general sense. It is critical to document, whenever possible, the duration of anemia; anemia of acute and recent onset, for exam-

TABLE 2–2.–PATHOPHYSIOLOGY OF ANEMIA

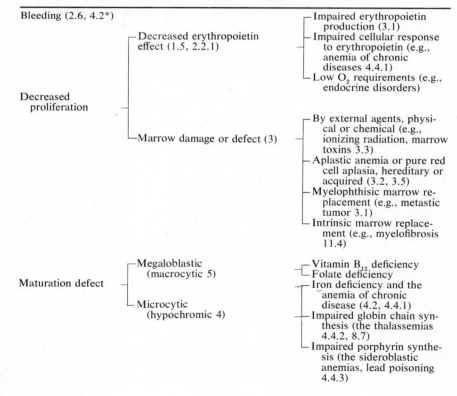

TABLE 2-2.—*(Continued.)*

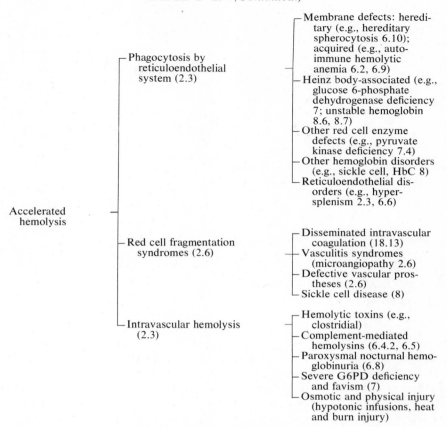

Accelerated hemolysis

- Phagocytosis by reticuloendothelial system (2.3)
  - Membrane defects: hereditary (e.g., hereditary spherocytosis 6.10); acquired (e.g., autoimmune hemolytic anemia 6.2, 6.9)
  - Heinz body-associated (e.g., glucose 6-phosphate dehydrogenase deficiency 7; unstable hemoglobin 8.6, 8.7)
  - Other red cell enzyme defects (e.g., pyruvate kinase deficiency 7.4)
  - Other hemoglobin disorders (e.g., sickle cell, HbC 8)
  - Reticuloendothelial disorders (e.g., hypersplenism 2.3, 6.6)

- Red cell fragmentation syndromes (2.6)
  - Disseminated intravascular coagulation (18.13)
  - Vasculitis syndromes (microangiopathy 2.6)
  - Defective vascular prostheses (2.6)
  - Sickle cell disease (8)

- Intravascular hemolysis (2.3)
  - Hemolytic toxins (e.g., clostridial)
  - Complement-mediated hemolysins (6.4.2, 6.5)
  - Paroxysmal nocturnal hemoglobinuria (6.8)
  - Severe G6PD deficiency and favism (7)
  - Osmotic and physical injury (hypotonic infusions, heat and burn injury)

*The numbers in parentheses refer to sections of the text in which a discussion relevant to each mechanism of anemia may be found. Where no reference is provided, the discussion lies outside the scope of this introductory text.

ple, has completely different implications than a life-long congenital anemia or recurrent episodes of hemolysis. The history must elicit evidence relating to excessive blood loss, including a detailed menstrual history; evidence of melena; bright red blood in or on stools; hematemesis; hematuria or dark or red urine.

A review of exposure to medications and potentially harmful industrial or household toxins is always indicated. This must include any medications administered as a prior attempt to treat the anemias including iron, vitamins and proprietary remedies that may contain hematinic agents, as well as other drugs that may themselves be implicated in the etiology of anemia. Every drug or component of a compound medication must be identified and its potentialities assessed. A careful evaluation of the contribution of alcoholic beverage to the patient's diet is an unfortunate but essential part of an anemia workup for members of all socioeconomic groups. Drugs and toxins may produce anemia by a variety of mechanisms including:

1. Direct suppression of erythropoiesis (e.g., chloramphenicol, phenylbutazone).

2. Disordered erythroid cell maturation (e.g., diphenylhydantoin, alcohol).

3. Accelerated hemolysis (e.g., sulfa drugs

TABLE 2–3.–SIGNS AND SYMPTOMS
OF ANEMIA

Cardiorespiratory-Vascular
  Exertional dyspnea, tachycardia, palpitation, angina,
    claudication, orthopnea
  Bounding arterial pulses, capillary pulsation, vascular
    bruits, cardiac enlargement, murmurs, dependent
    edema, urinary frequency, nocturia
  Increased depth and rate of respiration
  Hemorrhagic lesions in the optic fundi
Neuromuscular
  Headache, vertigo, faintness, tinnitus
  Loss of concentration, fatigue, cold sensitivity
Skin
  Pallor, particularly of the mucous membranes, nail-
    beds, palm lines
  Delayed wound healing
Gastrointestinal
  Anorexia, nausea, flatulence, constipation, diarrhea
Genitourinary
  Menstrual irregularity, amenorrhea, menorrhagia
  Loss of libido or potency

or aspirin in genetically susceptible individuals; penicillin, α-methyldopa).

2.6 Laboratory Tests

Subsequent sections will elaborate on special aspects of diagnostic hematology and on laboratory studies designed to reveal specific hematologic defects. At this point, we shall only outline some of the initial steps in the laboratory analysis of an anemia — steps essential in establishing a mechanism and in ordering the probabilities in the differential diagnosis. There are at least three elements of this first appraisal of an anemia:

1. *Is there bleeding?*

Major acute hemorrhage generally is obvious; chronic low grade bleeding into the gastrointestinal tract or excessive menstrual blood loss may go unnoticed by the patient. Examination of several stool specimens for blood (hematest or guaiac test) is a necessary part of the evaluation of anemia. Chronic blood loss probably will be associated with the depletion of iron stores and production of iron deficiency (see Chapter 4).

Acute hemorrhage results in immediate contraction of the total circulating blood volume; the attendant symptoms and signs largely reflect the body's homeostatic cardiovascular responses to acute circulatory volume depletion. The symptoms and signs depend both upon the magnitude of the hemorrhage and upon the patient's underlying cardiovascular status. Anemia per se will not be detected by the usual laboratory tests for several hours since plasma and red cells are lost proportionately. Initial restitution of blood volume is by influx of extravascular tissue fluid and may take several days following a single acute hemorrhage. Hemoglobin, Hct and red cell values will fall progressively during this readjustment. Replenishment of the circulating red cell mass is almost exclusively by the production of new erythrocytes, a process that may take considerable time even when the erythropoietic tissues are normal and capable of optimal response to the stress of anemia.

2. *What are the relative contributions of production defects, accelerated hemolysis and ineffective erythropoiesis?*

Judicious interpretation of the reticulocyte count, serum unconjugated bilirubin, haptoglobin level and erythropoietic activity of the marrow may be entirely sufficient for the initial appraisal. The ^{51}Cr life span generally is reserved for the resolution of conditions with obscure and complex pathophysiology.

3. *What does evaluation of red cell morphology show?*

Red cell morphology provides a valuable guide to the differential diagnosis of anemia. Certain characteristic findings may be virtually diagnostic of specific disorders. The morphology of normal red cells and the variations that fall within normal limits are best learned by diligent examination of many normal blood smears. This is an area of considerable importance and one in which physicians should be prepared to make responsible and accurate observations.

Significant variations from normal red cell morphology may be classified as (1) variations in size, (2) variations in hemoglobin content and (3) variations in shape. Common variations and the terms used to describe them are listed below.

Variations in size really refer to variations in red cell volume and this must be remembered when estimating red cell size by microscopy. Red cell diameter is only one dimension of cell volume. Red cell volume may, of course, be either smaller than normal *(microcytic)* or larger than normal *(macrocytic)*. Normal size is commonly called *normocytic*. An estimate of the average red cell volume (mean cell volume [MCV]) can be calculated from values of the Hct and RBC count.

$$MCV = \frac{Hct}{RBC\ (millions)} \times 10 \mu^3$$
e.g., Hct = 45%, RBC = $5 \times 10^6/mm^3$
$$MCV = \frac{45}{5} \times 10 = 90 \mu^3$$

The RBC count is the variable most affected by experimental error. The MCV is most reliable when the RBC is determined by electronic cell counters. Under these conditions, average normal MCV is $95 \pm 8 \mu^3$. Estimation of red cell size by microscopic examination of the stained blood smear is in some respects more informative than the calculated MCV. In particular, it is possible to recognize a small population of macrocytic (see Fig. 2–2, F) or microcytic (see Fig. 2–2, C) cells that is insufficient to alter the MCV. Indeed, the number of macrocytes in pernicious anemia (see Chapter 5), and especially the number of microcytes in hereditary spherocytic anemia (see section 6.10) may be borderline with respect to MCV and yet be unmistakable to the experienced microscopist.

The presence of a mixed population of cells of different sizes is termed *anisocytosis* and should be qualified by a specific descriptor (i.e., macrocytic, microcytic). Microcytosis, especially when associated with hypochromia, is very suggestive of defective hemoglobin synthesis (see Chapter 4). Mac-

rocytosis, unless due to unusually large numbers of reticulocytes (which are larger than the mature red cell), strongly suggests megaloblastic anemia (vitamin B_{12} or folic acid deficiency), although other causes are known (see Chapter 5).

Variations in hemoglobin content. An estimate of average hemoglobin content (mean cell hemoglobin [MCH])/red cell can be derived from values of blood hemoglobin concentration (Hb) and RBC.

$$MCH = \frac{Hb}{RBC\ (millions)} \times 10 pg/cell$$
e.g., Hb = 15 gm/100 ml, RBC
$$= 5 \times 10^6/mm^3$$
$$MCH = \frac{15}{5} \times 10 = 30\ pg/cell$$

The average normal MCH is 32 ± 2 pg/cell in the adult.

An index of mean cell hemoglobin concentration (MCHC) also can be calculated.

$$MCHC = \frac{Hb}{Hct} \times 100\ gm/100\ ml\ red\ cells$$
e.g., Hb = 15%, Hct = 45%
$$MCHC = \frac{15}{45} \times 100 = 33.3\ gm/100\ ml$$

The normal MCHC is 34 ± 2 gm% in adults. Red cell hemoglobin content, just as red cell volume, can and always should be estimated from examination of the stained smear. Normally hemoglobinized red cells are called *normochromic* (see Fig. 2–2, A). By comparison with normochromic cells, poorly hemoglobinized red cells are faintly stained, the central region of pallor is larger than normal and the cells appear thin. This condition is termed *hypochromia* (see Fig. 2–2, D). Hypochromic erythrocytes are usually microcytic. Disorders of hemoglobin synthesis including iron deficiency, thalassemia and sideroblastic anemias demonstrate hypochromia (see Chapter 4).

In addition to hemoglobin content, examination of the stained smear will reveal other tinctorial abnormalities of RBC. *Polychro-*

masia denotes a faintly bluish (basophilic) cast to the red cell (due to the RNA content of young erythroid cells); polychromasia implies a younger than normal population and may reflect an elevated reticulocyte count (a reticulocyte count must be performed to confirm this inference) or intense stimulation by erythropoietin. At times the basophilia may be punctate *(diffuse stippling)*, which has the same significance. *Coarse basophilic stippling* is seen in lead poisoning and ineffective erythropoiesis. *Howell-Jolly bodies* are small nuclear remnants; they are normally very rare, but increased numbers of cells containing a Howell-Jolly body are seen after splenectomy and in some severe hemolytic anemias.

Variations in shape. Poikilocytosis denotes variability of red cell shape, compared with the uniformity (smooth biconcave disks) of normal red cells (see Fig. 2–2, A and B). In itself, poikilocytosis is not diagnostic of any specific disorder but is observed in many conditions of disordered erythropoiesis or hemolysis. The qualifications *mild*, *moderate* or *marked* are generally added. It is informative to comment upon the presence of certain specific deformities, which, although not necessarily diagnostic, may be helpful in ordering the priorities in a complete evaluation. These include:

1. *Spherocytes,* round rather than discoid cells (see Fig. 2–2, C). Their transverse diameter is reduced due to sphering and loss of surface membrane. Spherocytes, often in small numbers, are characteristic of both inherited and acquired cell surface lesions (see Chapter 6).

2. *Leptocytes,* unusually thin, hypochromic red cells characteristic of disorders of hemoglobin synthesis such as thalassemia and severe examples of iron deficiency (see Fig. 2–2, D and E).

3. *Macro-ovalocytes,* the characteristic macrocyte of megaloblastic anemia. Frequently accompanied by hypersegmented granulocytes (see Fig. 2–2, F).

4. *Schistocytes,* sometimes described as "helmet-shaped" cells (see Fig. 2–2, G). Variable numbers of these fragmented cells may be seen in anemic states due to intravascular hemolysis, particularly when caused by disease involving the small blood vessels (microangiopathic hemolytic anemia) or malfunctioning vascular prosthetic devices.

5. *Nucleated erythrocytes* (NRBC), orthochromatic erythroblasts, normally confined to the marrow (see Fig. 2–1). They may be found in small numbers in the blood in many anemias but are particularly prevalent in myelosclerosis, in myeloid metaplasia with myelofibrosis (see section 11.4), in other causes of myelophthisis and in examples of severe, long-standing ineffective erythropoiesis such as thalassemia (see section 8.7).

6. *Target cells,* cells with a bull's-eye appearance due to a central concentration of hemoglobin within the zone of pallor (see Fig. 2–2, H). Target cells may be seen in many conditions of hypochromia and leptocytosis (thalassemia, severe iron deficiency); they are particularly frequent in hemoglobin C disease (HbC), but their presence in such nonhematologic disorders as acute and chronic liver disease attests to the nonspecificity of this finding.

7. *Sickle cells,* red cells that contain hemoglobin S, can be induced to undergo reversible distortion into bizzarre angular shapes due to hemoglobin tactoid formation (see Fig. 2–2, I). Various methods for inducing this deformation by deoxygenation provide the basis for certain laboratory screening tests for sickle cell syndromes.

8. *Teardrop-shaped poikilocytes,* highly suggestive of disordered marrow hematopoiesis such as myelophthisis or myeloid metaplasia (see Fig. 2–2, J).

9. *Acanthocytes,* cells with large, irregular, rounded, irreversible projections found in hereditary abetalipoproteinemia and acquired disorders of blood lipoproteins, as in liver failure.

3

Bone Marrow Failure

3.1 Introduction

ABSOLUTE OR RELATIVE failure of the bone marrow to produce adequate numbers of red cells contributes to the pathogenesis of anemia in a wide variety of clinical conditions (see Table 3–1 for a list of causes of marrow failure). Taken as a whole, such conditions comprise the bulk of the anemias. Marrow failure may involve a production defect at several levels of cellular development. When proliferating erythroblasts are present in significant numbers and yet reticulocytes fail to reach the blood stream, *ineffective erythropoiesis* is the mechanism of marrow failure, as previously described (see section 2.2.7.2). If, on the other hand, the marrow displays a paucity of proliferating erythroid precursors, the problem is *erythroid hypoplasia*. One mechanism for erythroid hypoplasia is decreased production of erythropoietin, which contributes to the anemia of renal insufficiency, to the anemia of chronic disease, to the anemias that accompany endocrinopathies with decreased metabolic demands and to the rare hemoglobinopathies with decreased oxygen affinity.

TABLE 3–1.—CAUSES OF BONE MARROW FAILURE

Aplastic anemia due to bone marrow suppression by chemical and physical agents

"Idiopathic" aplastic anemia, acute and chronic

Neoplastic disease involving marrow (primary or metastatic)

Congenital and familial aplastic states
    Congenital aplastic anemia
    Familial aplastic anemia with developmental anomalies (Fanconi type)

Metabolic or toxic bone marrow suppression secondary to other disease
    Chronic infection
    Rheumatoid arthritis
    Renal failure
    Endocrinopathies
    Neoplastic disease

Nutritional deficiency states: vitamin B_{12}, folic acid, pyridoxine, protein (due to dietary inadequacy or absorption defects); usually manifest as ineffective hematopoiesis

Hypoplastic-aplastic conditions predominantly affecting erythroid elements
    Pure red cell aplasia, associated with thymoma and other neoplasms; idiopathic
    Chronic erythrocytic hypoplasia
    Erythroid hypoplasia in hemolytic disease ("hypoplastic crisis")

"Primary refractory" anemias with cellular bone marrow

3.2 Pancytopenia and Aplastic Anemia

Injury to hematopoietic precursor cells or pluripotent stem cells, due to a variety of agents, is another cause of hypoproliferative anemia and commonly affects more than one of the marrow cell types. Pure red cell hypoplasia is uncommon. Generally, *pancytopenia* (reduced red cell, granulocyte and platelet concentrations in the blood) is the principal hematologic finding. Pancytopenia accompanied by generalized hypoplasia of the hematopoietic precursors is called *aplastic anemia*. Aplastic anemia is only one of a number of causes of pancytopenia; pancytopenia may result from destruction of circulating blood cells, as well as from production defects (Table 3–2).

3.2.1 CAUSES OF APLASTIC ANEMIA

Historically, chemical agents were the first recognized causes of aplastic anemia. Crude benzene (benzol) was the cause of many early cases due to widespread industrial exposure; carbon tetrachloride is another well-described industrial toxin. More sporadically the various insecticides have been implicat-

TABLE 3–2.—CAUSES
OF PANCYTOPENIA

Bone marrow failure (see Table 3–1)
Peripheral sequestration and destruction of circulating blood cells
    Hypersplenism (may occur in splenomegaly of any cause)
        Congestive splenomegaly
        Infection, infectious granuloma and inflammatory states: tuberculosis, sarcoid, histoplasmosis, syphilis, malaria, rheumatoid arthritis (the Felty syndrome)
        Metabolic disorders (the Gaucher, Niemann-Pick and Letterer-Siwe diseases)
        Lymphomas, chronic leukemia with complicating hypersplenism
    Autoimmune pancytopenia
    Microangiopathic hemolytic states, RBC and platelets affected principally)
Other primary hematologic disease, including megaloblastic anemia and paroxysmal nocturnal hemoglobinuria

ed. Currently the most common agents are pharmacologic rather than industrial. A list of the major drug-aplastic anemia reports is found in Table 3–3. Lists and data of this sort were regularly prepared by the Food and Drug Administration (*H.E.W. Bulletin: Clinical Experience Abstracts*). The incidence figures depend partly upon therapeutic patterns. In the preantibiotic era, organic arsenicals used in antiluetic therapy were a common offender. At present, the antibiotic chloramphenicol leads the report list. Other offenders among the common drug group are the anticonvulsants, especially the analgesic, phenylbutazone; the hypoglycemic, tolbutamide; the diuretic, acetazolamide and the sulfonamides.

The mechanism of damage inflicted by these agents, which unpredictably and sporadically produce severe marrow injury, is unknown. Several poorly defined possibilities have been suggested, including (1), a metabolic effect on cellular differentiation, and (2) an autoimmune mechanism directed against immature hematopoietic precursor cells and activated by the drug.

Unlike the low incidence of hematopoietic disease from these agents, hypoplasia may quite regularly be induced by certain chemical or physical agents designed for their cytotoxic actions. These include external x-irradiation, irradiation by incorporated isotopes (e.g., ^{32}P) or the various cytotoxic drugs employed in cancer chemotherapy. The use of such agents, which generally have low "therapeutic indices," is fraught with the hazard of marrow suppression.

3.2.2 CLINICAL PATTERNS

The response of patients exposed to chloramphenicol, the most frequently implicated drug at present, has been studied in some detail. Two response patterns have been described. The most common is an anemia that is dose related and is accompanied by reticulocytopenia in the circulation and by vacuolated erythroblasts in the marrow.

TABLE 3–3.—DRUGS ASSOCIATED WITH
APLASTIC ANEMIA*

AGENT	ALONE	TOTAL CASES (ALONE & COMBINED WITH OTHER AGENTS)
Antibacterials		
Chloramphenicol	179	322
Sulfamethoxypyridazine	3	14
Sulfasoxazole	3	29
Penicillin	4	100
Tetracyclines	4	94
Analgesics		
Phenylbutazone	18	40
Oxyphenbutazone	1	1
Acetylsalicylic acid	7	90
Phenacetin	3	33
Anticonvulsants		
Diphenylhydantoin sodium	3	23
Methyl-phenyl-ethyl-hydantoin	7	22
Trimethadione	3	6
Primidone	2	11
Hypoglycemics		
Tolbutamide	6	12
Carbutamide	1	2
Chlorpropamide	2	4
Diuretics		
Acetazolamide	3	10
Chlorothiazide	1	1
Antihistamines		
Chlorpheniramine	2	17
Tripelennamine	1	12
Insecticides		
Gamma-benzone hexachloride	10	17
Chlorophenothane (DDT)	3	21
Chlordane	0	12
Others		
Benzene	8	10
Quinacrine	3	5
Pyrimethamine	2	5
Meprobamate	0	12
Chlordiazepoxide	2	7
Gold compounds	8	10

*From Registry on Adverse Reactions, Council on Drugs, American Medical Association.

These lesions, and the anemia, revert to normal upon withdrawal of the antibiotic. Leukopenia and thrombocytopenia are rare, although myeloid precursors occasionally show toxic changes. The second and far less common manifestation is aplastic anemia following a variable and unpredictable dose of the antibiotic, which may appear even after the drug has been withdrawn. The clinical manifestations, as is typical of aplastic anemia in general, are the consequence of the duration, degree and extent of pancytopenia. Bleeding due to thrombocytopenia and infection secondary to granulocytopenia are compounded with anemia according to the severity of depression of each cell line.

The anemia of aplastic anemia is basically normocytic and normochromic and displays a markedly depressed reticulocyte count. Nucleated red cells and immature leukocytes in the circulating blood are distinctly unusual and their presence dictates a careful reappraisal of the differential diagnosis and a search for marrow invasion by both hematologic and nonhematologic neoplasms, granulomas or fibrosis. Hepatosplenomegaly is not common in aplastic anemia and, when observed, appears late in the course of the disease. Bone marrow aspiration is hypocellular, and it is often difficult to obtain a satisfactory diagnostic specimen by this technic. Needle biopsy reveals fatty replacement of normal architecture, interspersed in some specimens by zones of active marrow. The overall volume of effective marrow is strikingly reduced. Depressed erythropoiesis results in disturbed iron kinetics. Plasma iron content is elevated, and marrow iron stores are increased in the connective tissue and reticulum cells. Plasma iron clearance is low to normal, with iron delivery principally to nonmedullary (e.g., hepatic) reticuloendothelial tissues. Effective erythropoiesis, i.e., the reappearance of administered tracer iron in red cell hemoglobin, is markedly reduced.

The prognosis of aplastic anemia is guarded. In large series some 50% of patients die as a direct consequence of hemorrhage, infection or anemia; 20% require continued transfusions and perhaps 30% recover sufficiently to require no support, even though blood counts may remain abnormal indefinitely. A small but significant number of patients, after a variable period, develop overt acute myelogenous leukemia (see Chapter 10) or paroxysmal nocturnal hemoglobinuria (see section 6.8).

3.2.3 THERAPY

Treatment of aplastic anemia involves:

1. *Discontinuance of all potentially toxic agents* or drugs.

2. *Supportive management. Transfusion* for anemia must be used judiciously and only when the anemia causes real physiologic disability or when bleeding, usually due to platelet deficiency, is life threatening. Unneeded transfusion only increases the opportunity to develop immune reactions to platelets and to shorten the transfused life span of this formed element. *Platelet concentrates* may be transfused for life-threatening thrombocytopenia, but the emergence of antiplatelet antibodies may decrease their effectiveness. Careful attention to HL-A typing of donor platelets can alleviate but not eliminate the problem of isosensitization. *Adrenocortical steroids* may improve hemostasis in the presence of thrombocytopenia.

White cell transfusion can be used when efficient cell-separator equipment is available, but the logistics of this procedure, requiring large supplies of donor blood in order to provide only transiently effective circulating white cell levels, leaves this a relatively inefficient therapeutic modality. Infectious complications of the granulocytopenia of aplastic anemia are best handled by appropriate microbiologic studies and the use of judiciously selected antibiotic regimens, addressed as rapidly as possible to identified pathogens. Infection by opportunistic agents such as Listeria, Histoplasma, Aspergillus, Candida and Nocardia is of considerable clinical significance in these conditions. At extreme levels of granulocytopenia (under 500 cells/cu mm), isolation precautions are probably in order.

3. *Marrow stimulation.* Androgenic hormones have shown some promise in aplastic anemia, especially in children and when the marrow shows evidence of residual erythropoiesis. Prolonged (4–6 months) trials are indicated before failure is accepted. One documented effect of androgen is an enhanced release of erythropoietin, but this effect does not fully explain the apparent beneficial effects of androgens on hematopoiesis.

4

Disorders of Heme Synthesis: Iron Metabolism and Hypochromic Anemias

4.1 The Normal Steady State

THE BIOLOGIC REQUIREMENT for iron reflects almost exclusively the role of this metal in the porphyrin components of a variety of respiratory pigments (including hemoglobin for oxygen transport and the muscular respiratory pigment, myoglobin) and redox enzymes (cytochromes, cytochrome oxidase, xanthine oxidase, catalase, peroxidase, succinic dehydrogenase). About 70% of body iron is found in porphyrin molecules and the largest fraction is in hemoglobin. A normal adult male has a total body iron of about 4 gm. Of this, about 2.5 gm is in hemoglobin, 150 mg in myoglobin, 6–10 mg in respiratory enzymes, 3 mg in plasma transferrin and about 1 gm in the reticuloendothelial system as storage iron in the form of ferritin and hemosiderin (Fig. 4–1).

4.1.1 IRON TURNOVER

In normal males iron losses are about 1 mg daily, representing principally the iron contained in sloughed intestinal mucosal cells. Women, during the childbearing years, are subject to additional losses: 15 mg/month or more from menstrual blood loss and 600–800 mg at the time of each pregnancy. Iron balance is maintained by dietary replacement of these losses: about 1 mg daily is absorbed by normal men and twice this by normal adult women. It is apparent, however, that iron balance in women is more precarious than in men. Even in healthy, normally menstruating women, decreased reticuloendothelial iron stores may be found.

The internal turnover of iron reflects largely the marrow requirement for iron for replacement of effete red cells. Since the nor-

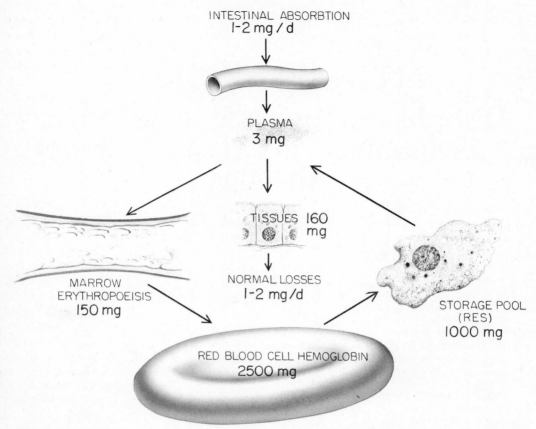

INTESTINAL ABSORBTION
1-2 mg / d

PLASMA
3 mg

TISSUES 160 mg

MARROW
ERYTHROPOEISIS
150 mg

NORMAL LOSSES
1-2 mg/d

STORAGE POOL
(RES)
1000 mg

RED BLOOD CELL HEMOGLOBIN
2500 mg

Fig. 4–1.— The distribution of iron in the several compartments of the body and the normal, steady state of iron absorption and loss. RES = reticuloendothelial system.

mal red cell life span is 100–120 days, about 0.8–1% of the circulating red cell mass (and hemoglobin) is destroyed and replaced daily, and 20–25 mg of iron a day must be provided to the erythropoietic tissues. This requirement is met almost exclusively by iron released in the spleen from aged red cells and transported to the marrow complexed with transferrin.

4.1.2 INTESTINAL ABSORPTION

Although the iron absorbed daily from dietary sources constitutes only a small fraction of the body iron pool, regulation of iron uptake in the intestine is a critical factor in iron homeostasis. Iron absorption can occur along the entire small intestine, but absorption is greatest in the proximal portions (duodenum) and falls distally. Under the mild alkaline conditions of the small intestine, ferrous iron and hemoglobin iron are more soluble and more readily absorbed than ferric iron. Food iron, however, is largely ferric in form; the absorption of dietary ferric iron is facilitated by chelation and complex formation in the acid stomach with amino acids, sugars and ascorbic acid, which solubilize the iron during its passage through the small intestine. The role of gastric hydrochloric acid in facilitating iron absorption may depend upon its ability to promote such soluble complex formation. The iron deficiency that at times accompanies gastrectomy or achlorhydria may occur on this basis.

An average daily U. S. diet contains some

10–20 mg of iron, of which 5–10% is absorbed (about 0.5–2 mg/day). Thus the intestinal mucosa normally rejects most of the iron presented to it. If increased amounts of iron are ingested, the quantity of iron absorbed increases, although the efficiency of absorption (proportion of ingested load absorbed) decreases. There is no absolute limit to iron absorption, and toxic, even fatal oral doses may inadvertently be ingested by children permitted unguarded access to medicinal iron preparations. The precise mechanisms that regulate the efficiency of intestinal absorption of ingested iron have yet to be fully elucidated. Early hypotheses, which postulated that saturation of mucosal apoferritin is the factor regulating intestinal iron transport, have not to date been validated experimentally and the nature of mucosal iron receptors or carriers remains problematic.

The efficiency of intestinal iron absorption increases physiologically in response to depletion of the body iron stores and decreases when erythropoiesis is suppressed and body iron is shifted into storage depots. The mediator regulating these responses at the absorptive surface is presently unknown. The efficiency of iron absorption also is increased under conditions of accelerated erythropoiesis even in the absence of reduced iron stores, as in the case of hemolytic anemias. Increased iron uptake under these conditions may lead to body iron overload, deposition of excess iron in various organs and tissue injury consequent to *secondary hemochromatosis*. The pathophysiology of *idiopathic hemochromatosis,* a familial condition in which there is continuous and accelerated intestinal iron absorption in the absence of anemia and in the face of progressive tissue overload, remains enigmatic.

4.2 Iron Deficiency States

4.2.1 CAUSES OF IRON DEFICIENCY

Blood loss is by far the most common cause of iron deficiency and iron deficiency anemia in the adult. The magnitude of the depletion attributable to blood loss is readily calculated: for every 100 ml of whole blood lost (containing 15 gm of hemoglobin), about 50 mg of iron is lost. Sites of pathologic blood loss include:

1. *Gastrointestinal.* This route must be thoroughly explored in any evaluation of iron deficiency, especially in the adult male or postmenopausal female. Gastrointestinal lesions to be considered include peptic ulceration, hiatus hernia, malignancies (particularly notorious are the often asymptomatic neoplasms of the cecum and of other portions of the large intestine and rectum), alcoholic gastritis, salicylate-induced gastric erosion, hookworm infestation and hemorrhoids.

2. *Gynecologic.* Excessive physiologic menstruation as well as menometrorrhagia secondary to intrinsic gynecologic pathology must be considered.

3. *Urinary tract.* Hematuria from kidney, ureter or bladder is a rare cause of iron deficiency. Chronic intravascular hemolysis at a rate sufficient to produce hemoglobinuria leads to hemosiderin deposition in renal tubular epithelial cells. Sloughing of these cells into the voided urine (hemosiderinuria) may lead to significant iron loss in the rare disorder, paroxysmal nocturnal hemoglobinuria, or in a patient with red cell fragmentation due to a malfunctioning prosthetic heart valve. Inadequate dietary intake of iron rarely is the sole or major cause of iron deficiency in Western societies except during infancy, the adolescent growth spurt or pregnancy. The normal full-term infant is born with moderate polycythemia and with iron stores adequate to see him through the first 4–5 months of life. After that the infant requires dietary iron for normal expansion of the red cell mass. Milk is a poor source of dietary iron, and supplements in the form of medicinal iron or fortified cereals may be required to maintain proper intake. Premature infants are particularly susceptible, since much of the placental transfer of iron from mother to fetus occurs in the latter weeks of pregnancy. During the period of rapid adolescent

growth, about 100–300 mg of extra iron/year is required and an inadequate diet may contribute to iron deficiency in this period. During pregnancy, although menses have ceased, sparing some blood loss, there are two demands on iron stores:

1. Iron loss with fetus (250 mg), with placenta (100 mg), and at delivery (75 mg).

2. A requirement for about 450 mg of iron that develops in the pregnant woman during the third trimester as her own red cell mass expands. Supplemental iron is advisable during pregnancy to cover these requirements.

Malabsorption may account for iron deficiency in the postgastrectomy state due to loss of the iron-solubilizing effect of hydrochloric acid as well as to physical bypass of the duodenal absorptive area. Marginal ulceration and bleeding must be excluded in the evaluation of postgastrectomy iron deficiency. Iron deficiency has been recognized at times in diffuse small intestinal disease and sprue syndromes. Iron-chelating compounds ingested in the so-called pica syndrome (compulsive starch or clay eating) may lead to iron deficiency. The role of these materials has yet to be fully evaluated since pica is also a well-recognized symptom of the iron-deficient state secondary to other causes.

4.2.2. Evolution of Iron Deficiency and Its Diagnosis

Negative iron balance induces a predictable sequence of events that develops in proportion to the severity of iron depletion:

1. *Progressive decline in reticuloendothelial iron stores*. Microscopic examination of the bone marrow stained with Prussian blue reagent provides a remarkably sensitive estimation of iron stores. In the presence of any stainable iron deposits in marrow, anemia cannot be attributed to iron deficiency since iron stores are fully exhausted before heme synthesis is compromised.

2. *Fall in concentration of plasma iron* and subsequently an elevation in plasma total iron binding capacity (TIBC, transferrin). The saturation of plasma transferrin (Fe/TIBC) consequently falls.

3. *Progressive anemia*, initially normocytic, normochromic, then microcytic and eventually microcytic and hypochromic, with variable degrees of poikilocytosis including elliptocytes and schistocytes. Reticulocytopenia is present throughout the evolution of the anemic stages of iron deficiency.

4. *Nonhematologic signs* of severe iron deficiency, including cheilosis, lingual depapillation, koilonychia, esophageal web, dysphagia and pica.

The diagnosis of iron deficiency anemia can be quite rigorously ascertained if this natural history is kept in mind. The requisite diagnostic criterion is the absence of storage iron in a marrow specimen. Development of microcytosis and hypochromia is not diagnostic; they are late manifestations of deficiency and also are found in other disorders due to defective hemoglobin synthesis, including the sideroblastic anemias, the anemia of chronic disease and the thalassemias. These all are associated with iron store overload rather than depletion.

4.3 Treatment of Iron Deficiency

There are two goals in the management of iron deficiency:

1. *To identify the cause* of the deficiency and to treat or remove that cause when possible. Since blood loss is the principal cause of iron deficiency, a thorough search for potential sites of blood loss is imperative.

2. *To correct the deficiency* by replenishment of body iron stores. Although achievement of this goal may provide immediate gratification to both patient and physician, it is only through a diligent and skillful search for a source of bleeding that the patient's best interests will be served.

Oral administration of water-soluble ferrous salts is the mainstay of iron replenishment; hydrated ferrous sulfate, 300 mg (60 mg elemental iron) three times daily, is the basic effective regimen. Mild gastrointestinal intolerance, manifested by diarrhea, constipation, nausea or epigastric discomfort, is a dose-related side-effect of medication and can be alleviated by dose reduction far more easily than by switching to alternative and generally more expensive iron preparations. Parenteral iron (intramuscular iron dextran) is reserved for patients in whom oral administration is impossible, unreliable or logistically infeasible.

When iron is given, reticulocytosis should occur within 7–10 days and a return to normal hemoglobin may be achieved within several weeks. Nevertheless, the goal of replenishment therapy is not only the return of hemoglobin to normal but the rebuilding of the depleted reticuloendothelial stores. The efficiency of iron absorption will be greatest initially (as much as 30–40 mg of elemental iron daily) and will fall progressively as iron storage improves. A rule of thumb dictates about 6 months of oral replenishment for severe iron deficiency anemia, assuming that the source of blood loss has been corrected.

Failure to respond to iron replacement suggests (1) continuing blood loss, (2) failure to take the oral preparation, (3) the wrong initial diagnosis or (4) malabsorption of medicinal iron. This last is an extremely rare situation and is a "last resort" explanation at best. If marrow iron stores remain empty (Prussian blue stain) and hypochromic anemia persists despite adequate oral supplement, parenteral iron may be administered as an alternative route.

4.4 Hypochromic Anemias in the Absence of Iron Deficiency

Anemia with variable degrees of hypochromia may be found in a number of disease states, both acquired and hereditary. Careful attention to the requisite diagnostic criteria should always permit accurate differentiation of these conditions from iron deficiency anemia. The principal discriminating feature is the presence or absence of stainable marrow iron stores. The main diseases in this group are the anemia of chronic disease, the thalassemias and the sideroblastic anemias.

4.4.1 ANEMIA OF CHRONIC DISEASE

A moderate and persistent anemia will develop in many patients suffering from chronic infections, inflammatory diseases (e.g., rheumatoid disease) or extensive neoplasia. The anemia may be normocytic and normochromic but not infrequently is hypochromic. The possibility of iron deficiency from chronic blood loss always must be considered under these circumstances and the role of contributory factors, such as aspirin ingestion, evaluated. In most cases, however, stainable marrow iron stores will be found adequate or increased despite red cell hypochromia and depressed serum iron levels. TIBC, unlike true iron depletion, is generally normal or depressed. There is, predictably, no hematologic response to medicinal iron.

The pathogenesis of the anemia of chronic disease is complex and not yet fully elucidated. A mildly accelerated rate of hemolysis (red cell life span of 80–90 days) is compounded by at least two additional pathogenic factors. In the first place, although tissue iron stores are replete, there is defective reutilization of iron released during the catabolism of effete red cells. Thus, the availability of iron for erythropoiesis is curtailed despite adequate storage iron. Secondly, in the face of chronic inflammatory states the production of erythropoietin is inadequate for the degree of anemia; thus the marrow fails to expand its erythropoietic capacity to meet the anemic stress. Evidence is also accumulating that indicates that the erythropoietic tissues also may show a somewhat refractory response even to the available erythropoietin.

4.4.2 THALASSEMIAS

Severe anemia with hypochromic, microcytic poikilocytosis is characteristic of the hereditary disorder of β chain globin synthesis, homozygous β-thalassemia (Cooley's anemia; see section 8.7.1). Marked hepatosplenomegaly, jaundice and retarded growth from early childhood are found; body iron stores are excessive and generally result in severe and life-threatening hemosiderosis (secondary hemochromatosis). Hypochromic poikilocytes in the presence of little or no anemia, absent or minimal organomegaly and a benign course are typical of the heterozygous form of β-thalassemia. Iron stores are adequate and the red cell morphologic abnormalities will not respond to iron. The diagnosis is based upon the presence of normal marrow iron in the face of the characteristic red cell changes, the family history, examination of blood smears from family members and the finding of an elevated hemoglobin minor component, HbA_2, in a majority of patients. The pathogenesis and clinical picture in these and related disorders of globin synthesis are discussed in a later section (see section 8.7).

4.4.3 Sideroblastic Anemias

The association of anemia with a mixed population of hypochromic and normochromic erythrocytes in the peripheral blood and with a prominent marrow population of erythroblasts containing deposits of stainable iron in mitochondria (so-called ringed sideroblasts because of the ring of iron granules disposed about the nucleus) characterizes the heterogeneous group of disorders termed the sideroblastic anemias. The common features in these disorders are the morphologic picture and disorder(s) of heme porphyrin metabolism leading to the accumulation of underutilized intraerythroblast iron. A considerable component of ineffective erythropoiesis is typical of these conditions.

The causes of sideroblastic anemia are varied and ill defined. A variety of toxic agents and drugs is associated with sideroblastic anemia. Of these, alcohol is by far the most frequent. The anemia of acute and chronic alcoholism exhibits a complex pathogenesis that may include blood loss, folate deficiency (with megaloblastic changes) and direct hematopoietic toxic effects including inhibition of normal heme synthesis and sideroblast formation. The anemia responds briskly to suspension of alcohol intake and to folate replacement. Thrombocytopenia and granulocytopenia also may be seen in acute alcoholism; the relative contributions of folate deficiency and direct toxic effects on hematopoietic precursors may not be easy to distinguish. Other toxic agents associated with sideroblastic anemia are chloramphenicol, lead, isoniazid, cycloserine and pyrazinamide.

A rare, genetically determined, sex-linked sideroblastic anemia in young males, which responds to long-term administration of large doses of pyridoxine, is reported. More commonly, "idiopathic" sideroblastic anemia develops without apparent cause in middle-aged to elderly patients, is refractory to all therapy including pyridoxine and may require transfusion therapy. The disorder generally culminates in death after a protracted course marked by progressive debility, infection, secondary hemochromatosis and, rarely, the onset of acute leukemia.

5

Megaloblastic Anemias

5.1 Introduction

THE MEGALOBLASTIC ANEMIAS are characterized by a spectrum of morphologic abnormalities of the nucleated hematopoietic precursors in the marrow and by severe ineffective erythropoiesis, often accompanied by ineffective leukopoiesis and thrombopoiesis. Additional manifestations, including neurologic disorders and abnormalities of the gastrointestinal epithelium, may accompany certain megaloblastic anemias, depending upon the etiology. The causes of megaloblastic anemia are listed in Table 5–1. Deficiencies of vitamin B₁₂ or of folate account for over 95% of the incidence of this anemia.

TABLE 5–1.—CAUSES OF
MEGALOBLASTIC ANEMIA

Vitamin B₁₂ deficiency
  Malabsorption
    Deficient intrinsic factor (IF)
      Pernicious anemia, acquired or congenital
      Total or partial gastrectomy
    Intestinal disorders
      Ileal resection
      Diffuse or patchy disease (Crohn's disease,
        tropical sprue)
      Fish tapeworm infestation
  Nutritional deficiency: vegan's diet
Folate deficiency or defective folate utilization
  Dietary: poor diet in old age, senility, chronic
    disease states, alcoholism
  Malabsorption
    Principal causes: tropical and nontropical sprue
    Drugs that interfere with or contribute to folate
      malabsorption: diphenylhydantoin, alcohol

Increased folate requirement or excessive losses
Pregnancy and lactation
Infancy, especially prematurity
Accelerated hematopoiesis, especially chronic
hemolytic anemias, sideroblastic anemias
Malignant diseases
Drugs that interfere with folate utilization:
antifolate agents used in treatment of neoplastic
diseases — methotrexate and aminopterin
Megaloblastic erythropoiesis independent of either
vitamin B_{12} or folate deficiency
Hematopoietic malignancies
Erythroleukemia and occasionally other leukemias
Sideroblastic anemias (some)
Orotic aciduria (hereditary)
Drugs that interfere with DNA synthesis, e.g.,
cytosine arabinoside, hydroxyurea

5.2 Clinical and Hematologic Manifestations

Macrocytosis, particularly macro-ovalo-cytes, with considerable poikilocytosis and anisocytosis; relative reticulocytopenia; neu-tropenia; thrombocytopenia and the pres-ence of hypersegmented neutrophilic granu-locytes represent the full-blown picture of megaloblastic anemia secondary to defi-ciencies of either of the two nutritional fac-tors, vitamin B_{12} and folate. The presence of hypersegmented neutrophilic granulocytes (more than five lobes) is reason enough, even as an isolated finding, to suggest B_{12} or folate deficiency, and further evaluation is indicat-ed. The marrow is hypercellular and displays evidence of disordered development of all three cell lines — erythroblasts, myeloblasts and megakaryocytes. The most prominent finding is megaloblastic maturation of the red cell series; the nucleus maintains a relatively primitive appearance despite progressive cytoplasmic maturation and hemoglobin syn-thesis. This morphologic manifestation, which includes a uniquely fine and lacy ap-pearance of nuclear chromatin, appears due to defective DNA synthesis. Nuclear frag-mentation is not uncommon and the intra-medullary destruction of many defective megaloblastic erythroblasts accounts for the prominent manifestations of ineffective erythropoiesis, including mild hyperbilirubi-nemia, elevated serum lactic dehydrogenase and erythroid hyperplasia without reticulo-cytosis. The granulocytic series displays giant precursor forms, especially notable at the metamyelocyte stage; megakaryocytes also are frequently enlarged and hyperpoly-ploid. The peripheral leukopenia and throm-bocytopenia despite adequate numbers of marrow precursors suggest that ineffective granulocytopoiesis and thrombocytopoiesis are part of the biologic effect of deficiency of vitamin B_{12} or folate.

Megaloblastic marrows respond rapidly to replacement with the deficient nutrient, so difficulties may be encountered in the inter-pretation of partially treated disease or fol-lowing improved diet. The term "megalo-blastoid," if used at all, should be confined to marrows in which erythroid cells display megaloblastic manifestations in the absence of vitamin B_{12} or folate deficiency; the granu-locytic and megakaryocyte stigmata usually are absent. "Megaloblastoid" marrows may be due to hematopoietic malignancies (erythroleukemias), sideroblastic anemias and certain rare congenital dyserythropoietic anemias. It should be noted that peripheral macrocytosis alone is by no means diagnos-tic of a megaloblastic anemia or of vitamin B_{12} or folate deficiency. Peripheral macrocy-tosis (elevated MCV) may be seen in myx-edema, liver disease, reticulocytosis of any cause or aplastic anemia. Finally, the mor-phologic manifestations of megaloblastic hematopoiesis are identical in both vitamin B_{12} and folate deficiency. Distinction be-tween them must be based upon other clini-cal features and upon specific laboratory studies.

5.3 Biologic Basis for Megaloblastic Anemia

It has already been noted that the megalo-blastic morphology is due to abnormal nucle-ar maturation and, in particular, to defective DNA synthesis. Both folate and vitamin B_{12}

participate in DNA production, as cofactors for the synthesis of critical deoxyribonucleotides, particularly the methylation of deoxyuridylate to form thymidylate (Fig. 5–1). This reaction requires N^5,N^{10}-methylene tetrahydrofolate to provide the methyl group for the thymidylate synthetase reaction. During transfer of the methyl group, tetrahydrofolate is oxidized to dihydrofolate, and an enzyme, dihydrofolate reductase, catalyzes the regeneration of tetrahydrofolate.

Thymidylate production and DNA synthesis are inhibited under a number of conditions, including (1) insufficient folic acid to form the active tetrahydrofolate, (2) inadequate conversion of folate to N^5,N^{10}-methylene tetrahydrofolate and (3) failure of reduction of dihydrofolate to tetrahydrofolate.

Folate deficiency due to dietary inadequacy, malabsorption or accelerated utilization undoubtedly affects DNA synthesis by the first mechanism. Certain antineoplastic chemotherapeutic agents (aminopterin and methotrexate) are powerful competitive inhibitors of the enzyme, dihydrofolate reductase. They cause megaloblastic transformation by inhibiting DNA synthesis by the third mechanism. Resistance to these agents

by neoplastic cells is associated with increased synthesis of dihydrofolate reductase.

Although the mechanisms described may account for the contribution of folate to DNA synthesis, the role of vitamin B_{12} in eukaryotic cells has not been completely elucidated. One hypothesis postulates a role for a vitamin B_{12} cofactor in the conversion of N^5-methyltetrahydrofolate to tetrahydrofolate and its metabolically active form, N^5,N^{10}-methylene tetrahydrofolate (the second mechanism of impaired DNA synthesis noted above). This reaction is linked with the B_{12}-dependent methylation of homocysteine to methionine. Failure of this reaction could explain the high levels of methyltetrahydrofolate observed in vitamin B_{12} deficiency. This putative mechanism for impaired DNA synthesis in vitamin B_{12} deficiency is commonly referred to as the "methylfolate trap" hypothesis.

5.4 Vitamin B_{12} Deficiency

Vitamin B_{12} malabsorption accounts for virtually the entire incidence of deficiency observed in the Western community. Vitamin B_{12} is synthesized solely by microorganisms and passed to man almost exclusively in food of animal origin. Dietary deficiency requires a strict vegan diet; this condition is achieved for religious reasons among strict Hindus, and dietary B_{12} deficiency is found in India. A typical Western diet, on the other hand, contains from $5-30$ μg of vitamin B_{12} daily. Normal body losses are between 1 and 3 μg/day, whereas total body stores average $2-3$ mg. Thus, even upon complete cut-off of supply (either from malabsorption or dietary reasons), B_{12} stores are adequate for $3-4$ years before manifest deficiency develops.

5.4.1 Intestinal Absorption and Transport

Vitamin B_{12} in reality comprises a family of so-called corrinoid molecules (the cobal-

Fig. 5–1.—Vitamin B_{12}, folate and the synthesis of DNA. dUMP = deoxyuridine monophosphate; dTMP = deoxythymidine monophosphate; FH_4 = tetrahydrofolate; FH_2 = dihydrofolate; NADP = nicotinamide adenine dinucleotide phosphate; NADPH = reduced NADP.

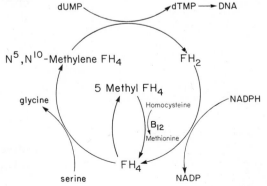

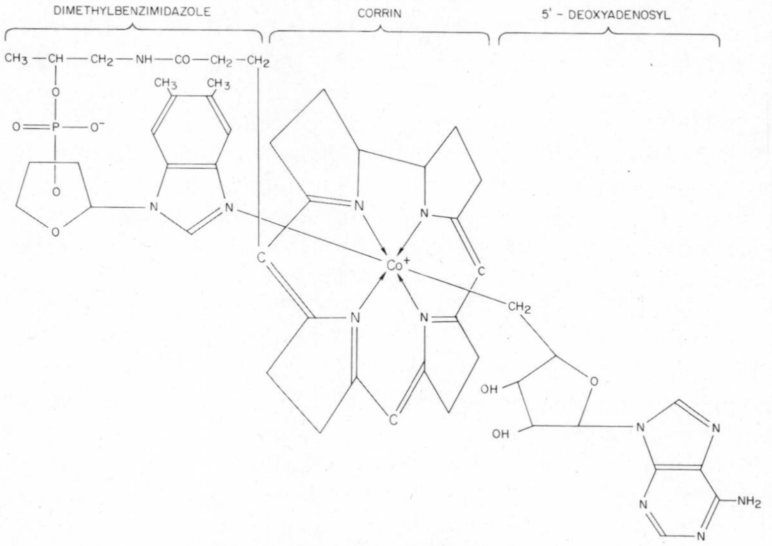

Fig. 5—2.—Structure of vitamin B_{12}.

amins) composed of a porphyrinlike moiety, liganded to cobalt (the corrin portion), and a nucleotide moiety (Fig. 5–2). Efficient absorption of vitamin B_{12} depends upon formation of a molecular interaction between cobalamin, liberated from food peptides by gastric proteases, and a glycoprotein called intrinsic factor (IF). IF is produced and secreted by gastric parietal cells. The IF-B_{12} complex attaches to specific receptor sites located exclusively on the ileal intestinal epithelium. Divalent cations and a neutral pH are required for attachment. The precise mechanism of transfer of vitamin B_{12} into and through the ileal mucosa is unknown, but IF is left behind. By about 6 hours after adsorption to the epithelium, labeled vitamin B_{12} can be found in the portal blood attached to a B_{12}-binding plasma protein, transcobalamin II.

Two major vitamin B_{12}-binding proteins are found in human plasma. Transcobalamin II, a β globulin with relatively low binding affinity, normally about 5% saturated with the vitamin, is the transport molecule, receiving cobalamin at the gut and delivering it at sites of utilization, including marrow. The bulk of plasma B_{12} is found on transcobalamin I, an α globulin with relatively high B_{12} affinity. Although transcobalamin I may be part of the body B_{12} storage pool, the precise role of this protein is unknown. Transcobalamin I is produced by granulocytic leukocytes, and the plasma level of this binding protein may be strikingly elevated in the presence of enlarged granulocyte pools and increased granulocyte turnover, such as in chronic myelogenous leukemia (CML). In vitamin B_{12} deficiency, transcobalamin I saturation falls and the level of plasma B_{12} (measured by either microbiologic or isotopic technics) decreases from a normal range of about 160–900 pg/ml to levels below 100 pg/ml.

5.4.2 INTESTINAL ABSORPTION (SCHILLING TEST)

A direct and extremely useful test of vitamin B_{12} absorption depends upon the urinary excretion of isotope-labeled vitamin B_{12} following oral administration (Schilling test). A small dose of ^{57}Co-labeled B_{12} is taken by mouth and shortly thereafter a large parenteral (intramuscular) injection of unlabeled B_{12} is given. The latter ensures that tissues and plasma are saturated with the vitamin. Urine is collected for 24 hours and assayed for excretion of the orally administered radioactive B_{12}. Following a 1 μg oral dose, normal subjects will excrete over 5% of the radioactivity within 24 hours. B_{12} malabsorption is indicated by low levels of excretion. Erroneously low excretion may be due to inadequate urine collection or to renal disease with poor glomerular filtration. It should be noted that the Schilling test involves administration of a large therapeutic dose of the vitamin; this must be kept in mind in designing a diagnostic strategy for any individual patient. Variants of the Schilling test include (1) administration of active hog gastric IF along with orally administered labeled B_{12} (Schilling "part II") to ascertain whether the low excretion in the standard Schilling test (Schilling "part I") is due to IF deficiency (pernicious anemia); and (2) repeat Schilling test after a period of orally administered antibiotics (Schilling "part III") to determine the role of altered intestinal bacterial flora in B_{12} malabsorption.

5.4.3 CLINICAL FEATURES

Clinical manifestations of B_{12} deficiency, including megaloblastic anemia, do not differ from those of folate deficiency save in the specific laboratory evidence of decreased plasma vitamin B_{12} levels and defective B_{12} absorption, and in one major clinical manifestation. B_{12} deficiency, but not folate deficiency, entails significant risk of severe neurologic disorder. The full-blown classic neurologic syndrome of vitamin B_{12} deficiency, subacute combined degeneration of the nervous system, consists of the following manifestations:

1. Peripheral neuropathy evidenced by paresthesias of fingers and toes.

2. Posterior column damage resulting in decreased position and vibratory sensation.

3. Lateral column damage with hyperactive deep tendon reflexes, spasticity and positive confirmatory toe signs.

4. Cerebral dysfunction, at times with manifestations of psychosis.

Not all of these need be present simultaneously. Reversibility upon vitamin replenishment is variable and unpredictable. Remarkably rapid clearance of cerebral dysfunction has been reported. The biochemical basis for the neurologic disorders remains obscure. It is well recognized, however, that inappropriate treatment of megaloblastic anemia due to B_{12} deficiency by large doses of folic acid may rectify the hematopoietic defect and yet precipitate severe and previously unrecognized neurologic disease.

5.4.4 MALABSORPTION DUE TO IF LACK (PERNICIOUS ANEMIA AND THE POSTGASTRECTOMY SYNDROME)

Pernicious anemia is the major cause of B_{12}-deficiency megaloblastic anemia in the Western community. The basic lesion is gastric atrophy and failure of IF secretion by parietal cells. It is invariably accompanied, in the adult onset form, by gastric achlorhydria. There is a rare childhood variant, inherited as an autosomal recessive gene, manifested by isolated IF deficiency without gastric atrophy or achlorhydria. The etiology of the gastric epithelial disorder in pernicious anemia is unknown, but familial incidence and association with disorder of one or another of a group of endocrine organs (thyroid, adrenal, pancreas) in some patients and their families suggests an as yet unrecognized hereditary mechanism.

The regular appearance in pernicious anemia of a number of abnormal immunologic phenomena — in particular antibodies to IF, to parietal cells and to thyroid antigens — raises the possibility of an autoimmune pathogenesis, but the actual role of immune mechanisms remains unclear.

Vitamin B_{12} deficiency will invariably follow total gastrectomy, when storage B_{12} is exhausted (generally by 3–4 years). B_{12} replacement is indicated following this surgical procedure. Following subtotal gastrectomy,

B_{12} deficiency and megaloblastic anemia also may occur, depending principally upon the extent of resection. Associated iron deficiency is common and both this and B_{12} deficiency may require continuous replacement therapy.

5.4.5 DIAGNOSIS OF PERNICIOUS ANEMIA

Diagnosis is based on the following factors:

1. The classic stigmata of megaloblastic anemia.

2. Evidence of neurologic disease, strongly indicative of B_{12} rather than folate deficiency.

3. Presence of histamine-fast achlorhydria. This is an essential component of pernicious anemia; however, since it may occur with advancing age in the absence of pernicious anemia, its presence is not sufficient to rule out other causes of megaloblastic anemia.

4. Direct evidence of B_{12} lack and B_{12} malabsorption.

This latter requirement can be met by the B_{12} plasma assay and the Schilling test, if available. When these are not accessible, it is still possible to distinguish B_{12} from folate deficiency by a therapeutic trial with physiologic doses ($1-2$ μg daily) of B_{12} given intramuscularly. This regimen will result in a therapeutic response (reticulocytosis in $5-7$ days, rising hemoglobin thereafter, conversion to a normoblastic marrow) in true vitamin B_{12} deficiency but not in folate deficiency. In a complementary fashion, physiologic doses of folate ($100-200$ μg daily by mouth or intramuscularly) will rectify folate but not B_{12} deficiency. This approach, although theoretically sound, must be considered cautiously in the elderly debilitated or in those with cardiovascular compromise in whom a prompt therapeutic response may be imperative. In any case, there is never an excuse to take unnecessary risks; serum samples may be drawn immediately and stored for subsequent B_{12} or folate assay, the Schilling test can be postponed (since in pernicious anemia it will remain diagnostic even after treatment) and full therapeutic doses of both B_{12} and folate may be given promptly even while awaiting a final diagnostic decision. Cautious transfusion of small amounts of packed red cells can be considered, but it must be recognized that these patients tolerate the cardiovascular load poorly and ensuring a gradual response to B_{12} replacement is generally a safer approach.

5.4.6 TREATMENT OF PERNICIOUS ANEMIA

Long-term therapy of pernicious anemia requires replenishment of body B_{12} stores and a maintenance regimen sufficient to supply the $2-5$ μg of B_{12} needed daily. A reasonable program is 100 μg intramuscularly daily for about 2 weeks, followed by monthly injections of 100 μg for life. Larger doses for the first $4-6$ months should be used to insure maximal recovery in the presence of neurologic manifestations. Iron therapy is not regularly required, since iron stores in megaloblastic anemia usually are replete or even excessive. Occasional patients have a concomitant borderline iron store, which only becomes an overt deficiency during the B_{12}-induced remission. A suboptimal reticulocytosis and hemoglobin rise accompanied by some hypochromia may provide a clue to associated iron deficiency, which should be confirmed and treated as already described (see section 4.3). Finally, the incidence of gastric carcinoma is significant among patients developing pernicious anemia. An initial upper gastrointestinal x-ray series followed by regular monitoring of gastrointestinal symptomatology and the stool hematest for occult bleeding is indicated.

5.4.7 MALABSORPTION OF VITAMIN B_{12} DUE TO INTESTINAL CAUSES

Malabsorption of vitamin B_{12} due to intestinal disorder may be observed in two basic situations:

1. Defective ileal absorbing surface, either nonspecific (due to surgical resection, regional ileitis, tropical and nontropical sprue with ileal involvement) or specific for IF-B_{12} binding sites (due to congenital B_{12} malabsorption, the Imerslund-Grasbek syndrome).

2. Competitive destruction of B_{12} by abnormal bacterial flora or parasites resident in the upper intestine, often in relation to anatomic abnormalities (strictures, diverticula, anastomoses and blind loops due to surgical procedures). It is postulated but not definitively proved that the abnormal bacteria found under these circumstances ingest vitamin B_{12} and prevent ileal absorption. A similar interpretation is offered for the vitamin B_{12} deficiency that may accompany infestation with the fish tapeworm *Diphyllobothrium latum*.

In each of these conditions the Schilling test part II will be abnormal, i.e., the addition of exogenous IF will not correct the malabsorption. Additional studies to pinpoint the cause of malabsorption may be useful, including Schilling test part III, bowel x-ray studies and other tests of malabsorption (fecal fat, D-xylose absorption, jejunal biopsy). Remedy of the malabsorption must be tailored to the nature of the intestinal defect.

5.5 Folate Deficiency

Folic acid, pteroylglutamate, is the parent compound of a family of closely related compounds, referred to collectively as the folates. The molecule contains three chemical moieties (Fig. 5–3): a pteridine residue, a *p*-aminobenzoic acid residue and either a single or multiple glutamate(s) linked by γ-peptide bonds (the pteroylpolyglutamates). Folates are found widespread in natural foods including green vegetables, fruits, liver, kidney and other sources. In nature the principal folates are pteroylpolyglutamates, partly or completely reduced in the pteridine portion to the di- and tetrahydrofolate form and bearing a one-carbon substituent such as

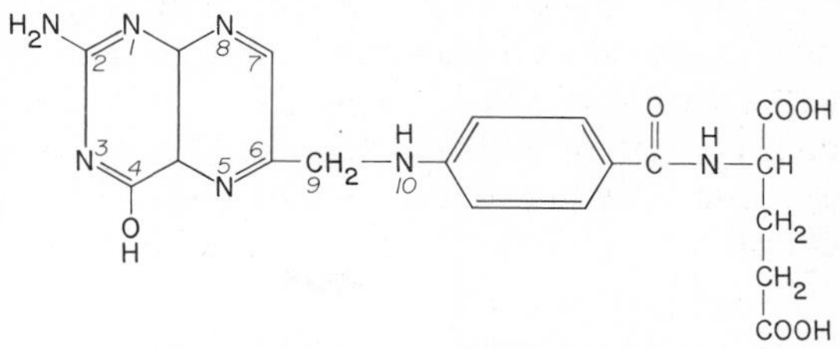

Fig. 5–3. — Structure of folic acid.

formyl, methyl or methylene groups. An average Western diet contains as much as 600 μg of folate, but this value varies considerably depending on food habits. Food folate levels are markedly reduced by excessive cooking.

Body folate stores are from 5–10 mg, at least one third of which is hepatic. Daily adult requirements are between 50 μg and 100 μg; storage folate can suffice only for about 4 months in the absence of dietary intake. Unlike vitamin B_{12}, interference with adequate folate intake can lead rapidly to severe deficiency and megaloblastic anemia.

5.5.1 ABSORPTION

Folate absorption is maximal in the proximal small intestine (duodenum and jejunum) and falls off progressively at distal sites. Absorption is rapid and the intestine has a high capacity for folate uptake. Folic acid, the usual therapeutic folate, is more efficiently absorbed than the conjugated polyglutamate forms found in foodstuffs. These latter compounds undergo enzymatic hydrolysis to the monoglutamate during or prior to absorption. The metabolic conversion of folic acid to the active coenzyme, N^5,N^{10}-methylene tetrahydrofolate, has already been described (see section 5.3).

5.5.2 DIAGNOSTIC FEATURES

The clinical diagnosis of folate deficiency is based upon the following:

1. Hematologic evidence of megaloblastic anemia (indistinguishable from that secondary to B_{12} deficiency).

2. Presence of characteristic clinical syndromes associated with folate deficiency.

3. Specific studies designed to distinguish folate deficiency from B_{12} malabsorption, principally serum folate and B_{12} assay, or a therapeutic response to physiologic doses of folic acid (100–200 μg daily).

5.5.3 SPECIFIC CAUSES OF FOLATE DEFICIENCY

An outline of the major causes of folate deficiency is provided in Table 5–1. Dietary folate deficiency is not uncommon among patients prone to poor eating habits, including the elderly, senile, edentulous, alcoholic or chronically ill. Intestinal malabsorption of folate is characteristic of nontropical sprue and is reversed by a gluten-free diet. Tropical sprue is likewise accompanied by significant folate malabsorption; remarkably, the intestinal lesions of tropical sprue may be dramatically improved by folate administration despite the lack of evidence for insufficient folate in the diets of patients with tropical sprue. The basic pathogenesis of this disorder has yet to be satisfactorily elucidated.

Defective absorption of folate also has been ascribed to the administration of a number of therapeutic agents, most notably the anticonvulsant, diphenylhydantoin. Isoniazid and cycloserine also have been implicated in this regard. The mechanisms involved in folate malabsorption due to these agents have not been established.

Folate deficiency not infrequently becomes manifest when there is an augmented metabolic demand for this nutritional factor. Such circumstances are common because of the marginal supply of folate even in many normal diets. Pregnancy is probably the commonest of these situations; folate requirements increase to over 300 μg daily due to fetal demands. Deficiency is most likely during the last trimester. Multiple pregnancy, poor diet and lactation augment the severity of pregnancy-induced deficiency, and folic acid supplementation is a reasonable practice during pregnancy. Chronically hyperactive hematopoiesis, particularly the erythroid hyperplasia of sustained hemolytic anemia, also may precipitate folate deficiency. Relatively high doses of folic acid may be required to correct megaloblastic changes under these circumstances. Regular prophylaxis with folic acid is customarily given to patients with hereditary or unremitting hemolysis to avoid this complication. The megaloblastic state and depressed serum folate that may occur in widespread malignant disease may be explained on a similar basis.

It already has been pointed out that an important group of antineoplastic agents, the 4-aminopteroyl glutamates (aminopterin and methotrexate), act as powerful competitive inhibitors of the enzyme, dihydrofolate reductase, required for the generation of coenzymatically active tetrahydrofolate. These agents can produce megaloblastic anemia among their cytotoxic effects. N^5-formyl tetrahydrofolate ("citrovorum factor") can circumvent inhibition of the reductase; so-called "citrovorum rescue" may be provided when massive doses of methotrexate must be administered in a cancer chemotherapy protocol.

6

Hemolytic Anemia: Injuries at the Red Cell Membrane

6.1 Introduction

THE ERYTHROCYTE MEMBRANE is a dynamic structure, chemically complex and containing components responsible for a wide variety of functional properties. Structural complexity has become increasingly evident as newer ultrastructural technics have been brought to bear on red cell membrane. A model of membrane structure, which accounts for much of our present knowledge of membrane components and properties, is illustrated in Fig. 6–1. This model accommodates both a lipid bilayer and intercalated proteins and glycoproteins in the final membrane structure.

43

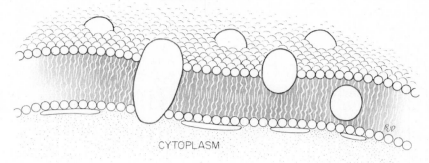

Fig. 6–1. — Model of cell surface structure. The membrane is conceived as a mosaic of proteins embedded in a lipid matrix. Some proteins span the entire membrane; others are at the surface or are fully embedded within the membrane. One protein, spectrin, is found just beneath the membrane of red blood cells. Mobility of the proteins in the membrane may depend, in part, upon their relationship both to the lipids and to other proteins.

Our knowledge of the chemical composition of the membrane is based primarily on analysis of red cell stroma, the material that remains after hemolysis and exhaustive washing to remove hemoglobin and other soluble proteins. The stroma consists of approximately 40–50% protein, 35–45% lipid and 5–15% carbohydrate. The lipid composition includes neutral lipids, glycolipids and glycolipoproteins. The mature erythrocyte does not synthesize lipids de novo, but several lipid components will exchange with lipids of the plasma. The rates of exchange are determined by a variety of factors including the relative concentrations of different lipid components in plasma and in the red cell. The proteins of the red cell membrane also are not well characterized. There appear to be at least a dozen red cell membrane proteins. Among these, two are major components: spectrin, which accounts for approximately 20% of the stromal proteins, and glycophorin, which accounts for about 10% of the membrane proteins. It is believed that glycophorin carries the A-, B-, M- and N-specific blood group antigens, as well as receptors for viruses and other surface-reactive substances. Whereas spectrin is located exclusively at the inner, cytoplasmic side of the membrane, glycophorin lies in part at least at the outer surface and may extend across the entire thickness of the red cell plasma membrane.

Accelerated hemolysis due to abnormalities at the red cell membrane may be acquired or hereditary. Injuries mediated by the immune system and by hereditary spherocytosis will be considered as paradigms of acquired and hereditary membrane lesions.

6.2 Immune Mechanisms

The interaction of antibodies with circulating RBC can result in hemolytic disease by a variety of mechanisms. Few of these mechanisms are as yet fully understood. Nevertheless, many of the factors that contribute to the nature and severity of immunologically mediated red cell disease have been identified, and their roles in the pathogenetic processes are becoming evident. What has become eminently clear in recent years is (1) that the interaction of immunoglobulin (Ig) with red cell surface antigens is not in itself sufficient explanation for many instances of hemolytic disease; and (2) that in vitro red cell-antibody reactions (whether simple hemagglutination, complement-mediated reactions or the now classic antiglobulin [Coombs] test), although informative, indeed critical, in the diagnosis of immune hemolytic disorders, do not in themselves provide a proper model capable of fully explaining the pathogenesis of hemolysis in vivo.

Among the factors that must eventually be included in an overall explanation of immune hemolytic diseases are the following:

1. The *nature of red cell antigens* implicated in the immune reaction. The chemical nature of the antigen and its relationship to structural and functional elements of the red cell membrane, the density and topographic distribution of antigenic sites and the effects of temperature and perhaps other as yet unrecognized environmental factors—all contribute to the clinical manifestations of immune reactions at the erythrocyte surface (see section 6.3).

2. The *nature of the antibody* involved in the immune reaction, including the biologic differences between IgG and IgM antibodies, the several IgG subclasses (IgG 1, 2, 3, 4) and other factors that affect the kinetics of antibody antigen reactions (see section 6.4).

3. The *role of non-Ig components* of the immune reaction, most particularly the complement and properdin systems, in mediating immune red cell injury (see section 6.5).

4. The interaction of antibody-injured red cell with each of the several organized units of the *reticuloendothelial system,* especially the spleen and liver (see section 6.6).

6.3 Red Cell Antigens

Red cell surface antigens may be polysaccharide (probably glycolipids or complex glycolipoproteins), protein or perhaps lipoprotein in structure. The red cell antigens are determined genetically, but the mechanism of expression differs according to the nature of each of the antigenic systems. In the case of polysaccharide-determined antigens (e.g., the ABO system), the effective gene products are glycosyl transferases capable of forming the specific glycosidic linkages that characterize each of the polysaccharide antigens. In the case of protein or lipoprotein antigens (the Rh system is considered to be of this sort), the gene product probably is the antigenic molecule itself.

6.3.1 ABO, H AND LEWIS SYSTEMS

Clinically the ABO system is the most significant of the blood groups. A and B antigenic activity, found on many if not all tissues including erythrocytes, also may be found in many body fluids. These antigens must be considered not only in blood transfusion but in all transplantations and during pregnancy. These antigens, or very closely related polysaccharide structures, are so common in nature that immunization to A or B antigens occurs very early in the life of individuals lacking either one or both. By tradition, antibodies so-formed are often called "natural" antibodies. The usual natural anti-A or -B antibodies are IgM in type, although some individuals, especially of type O, produce IgG anti-A and anti-B, in addition. This may be an important factor in the pathogenesis of erythroblastosis fetalis (see section 6.9).

The ABO system comprises two antigens, A and B, determined by two codominant alleles at the ABO genetic locus, which code for specific transferases that attach either N-acetyl-α-D-galactose (for A activity) or α-D-galactose (for B activity) in a 1→3 glycosidic linkage with the terminal β-D-galactose residue on a blood group precursor molecule with so-called H specificity (Fig. 6–2). Failure to produce both transferases, due to homozygosity for recessive transferase-negative alleles at the ABO locus, results in type O antigenicity. Thus, the O gene is considered an amorphic locus. Heterozygosity at the ABO locus (A/B; A/O; B/O) results in the anticipated antigenic phenotypes (AB; A; B). A and B structures, when present, are

Fig. 6–2.—Reactions that generate blood group-specific antigens.

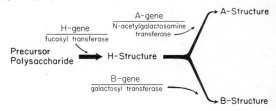

demonstrable in large numbers on the cell surface; 250,000 – 1,000,000 copies of A can be detected on type A red cells.

The H structure, determined by an independently segregating genetic locus, is determined by a transferase that places a fucose residue in 1→2 linkage to the terminal β-D-galactose of a precursor polysaccharide. The H structure is the substrate for addition of A or B antigens; the rare h/h genotype (so-called Bombay type), lacking any H-specific transferase, also lacks both A and B activity no matter what the genotype at the ABO locus.

Another independent genetic locus, secretor, with two alleles, Se and se, determines whether A, B and H antigenic activities are generated upon soluble mucopolysaccharides such as are found in saliva, gastric juice or amniotic fluids. The homozygous recessive se/se cannot place A, B or H in these fluids but does not interfere with their expession on cell surfaces.

Allelic variants of A and B transferase activity are known. One of these differs functionally in the K_m (Michaelis-Menton constant) of the enzyme and results in the antigenically weak expression of A activity known as A_2.

Lewis blood group activity (Le^a and Le^b) is related structurally to the ABO system but differs in being a soluble, plasma-borne antigenic material that attaches to, but is not a product of, the red cell membrane. Lewis activity is the product of a structural gene, segregating independently of the ABO and H loci, for a transferase that places α-L-fucose in 1→4 glycosidic linkage to N-acetyl-glucosamine on a precursor polysaccharide. Le is a dominant character; only the homozygous recessive le/le fails to generate this activity. The antigenic product of Lewis transferase activity is termed le^a and can be recognized by specific anti-le^a antisera. In the presence of the dominant gene Se, the H transferase (another fucosyl transferase; see above) is also active on soluble (e.g., plasma) polysaccharides; insertion of both the le-de-

termined fucose and the H-determined fucose generates soluble le^b antigenic activity, which, like le^a, binds to circulating red cell membranes.

6.3.2 RH SYSTEM

The clinical importance of the Rh system lies not in the presence of natural antibodies, as in the case of the ABO system, but rather in the ease with which an Rh-negative individual will form anti-Rh antibodies following mismatched transfusion with Rh-positive blood or following an Rh-incompatible pregnancy. The Rh blood type system, unlike the ABO-H group, is restricted to erythrocytes and is determined by a highly complex system of perhaps hundreds of alleles at several very closely linked genetic loci expressing over 30 antigenic variants. Despite the antigenic and genetic complexity of the system, Rh activity is represented at the red cell surface by far fewer antigenic sites than is the ABO system. It has been calculated that the Rh system controls only some 10,000 – 40,000 antigenic sites on the red cell membrane, depending on the genotype. Antibodies generated against Rh antigens following mismatched transfusion or Rh-incompatible pregnancy or in certain autoimmune hemolytic states are of the IgG class. IgG antibodies, unlike IgM, are transported across the placenta and can participate in the destruction of Rh-incompatible fetal red cells in the pathogenesis of erythroblastosis fetalis.

From a clinical point of view, Rh positivity refers to the presence of a particularly immunogenic and prevalent Rh antigen (Rhl, Rho or D according to the three most popular nomenclature systems); Rh-negative individuals lack this antigen. Our present understanding of the Rh system, since its discovery in 1939 by Levine and Stetson from a clinical observation and in 1940 by Landsteiner and Wiener from experimental studies, has been the result of painstaking accumulation of specific antisera that identify the individual antigenic components of the system. The simplest of the Rh notation systems designates antigens generated by three very closely linked genetic loci, called CDE, and their principal allelic alternatives, cde. Antisera are available that recognize gene products C, c, D, E and e. No substance with d activity has been identified and this gene apparently is expressed as the absence of D. Rh gene frequencies vary widely around the world. The commonest gene patterns in white and oriental populations are CDe (Weiner's R^1), cde (r) and cDE (R^2), to which in black populations must be added cDe (R^0). These complex gene patterns account for over 90% of the incidence of Rh genes; diploid combinations of these linked gene sets provide the commonly observed genotypes, e.g., Rh-positive: CDe/cde, CDe/CDe, CDe/cDE, cDE/cde and cDe/cDE; Rh-negative: cde/cde. Many other Rh alleles and combinations of alleles with very low gene frequencies are recognized.

6.3.3 OTHER SIGNIFICANT RED CELL ANTIGENIC SYSTEMS

Other blood antigens that have been implicated in clinical problems (e.g., erythroblastosis fetalis, transfusion reactions, autoimmune disease) include:

1. Duffy (fy) and Kidd (JR), which resemble ABO antigens in their genetic expression.

2. MN, a set of sialic acid-containing antigens present in high density at the cell surface.

3. Kell, comprising four sets of alternative alleles with amorphic genes as well, and responsible for both severe transfusion reactions and erythroblastosis fetalis.

4. Ii, the antigens implicated in most of the cold hemagglutinin disorders mediated by IgM autoantibodies, including chronic cold hemagglutinin disease and infectious mononucleosis. Cord blood is highly reactive with anti-i antisera; i-activity decreases and I-activity increases with normal maturation.

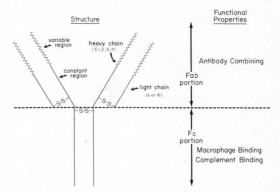

Fig. 6–3.—Basic immunoglobulin structure and functional properties.

The antigens I and i may bear a structural relationship to the A, B and H antigens.

6.4 Anti-Red Cell Antibodies

Antibodies active against RBC antigens have been detected among Ig of IgG, IgM and IgA types. Most clinically significant patterns of immune red cell injury can be ascribed to IgG and IgM activity, and our discussion will be confined to these classes. The basic Ig structure is illustrated in Fig. 6–3. The antigen-binding sites are located at the amino-terminal, variable-region end of the molecule in the so-called Fab fragment.

Fig. 6–4.—The IgM molecule, a pentamer of the basic immunoglobin molecule.

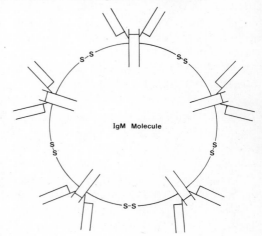

IgG and IgM each carry common light chains (with two classes, λ and κ) and unique heavy chains (γ, with subtypes γ^1, γ^2, γ^3, γ^4 for IgG; μ, with subtypes μ^1 and μ^2 for IgM). As illustrated in Figure 6–3, IgG is a monomeric Ig with two antigen-combining sites, whereas IgM (Fig. 6–4) exists as a pentamer of the basic Ig structure, displaying 10 antigen-combining sites.

The significant biologic properties of Ig are not confined to the antigen-binding capacity of the Fab fragment. The other portion of the molecule, the Fc fragment, also carries functional properties of great importance to the biology of immune reactions and to the pathogenesis of hemolytic disease. Among these are macrophage and complement binding.

6.4.1 ABILITY TO BIND SPECIFICALLY TO MACROPHAGES OF RETICULOENDOTHELIAL SYSTEM

This property is confined to IgG1 and IgG3 and is absent from IgM and the other IgG subclasses. RBC sensitized by antibodies with this characteristic can adhere to macrophages during passage through the spleen; adherent red cells are subject to complete or partial phagocytosis. Partial phagocytosis of bits of red cell membrane and cytoplasm causes sphering, which in turn renders the injured spherocyte liable to permanent sequestration by the spleen and to hemolysis by erythrophagocytosis.

6.4.2 ABILITY TO BIND COMPLEMENT COMPONENTS AT RED CELL MEMBRANE

This in turn leads either to adhesion of complement-bearing red cells to macrophages or to activation of the complete complement pathway and intravascular hemolysis. Many IgM and IgG antibodies will bind complement to red cell surfaces, but the several classes of Ig differ widely in their efficiency in this regard. IgM is, over-all, much the most efficient in complement binding; IgG1, IgG3 and IgG2 display progressively decreasing complement-binding ability and IgG4 has no apparent activity. The specific role of complement in immune hemolysis is dealt with in more detail below (see section 6.5).

6.4.3 THERMAL PROPERTIES OF ANTIBODIES

Red cell-reactive antibodies also may be distinguished by the optimum temperature at which they bind to red cell antigens. Cold-reactive antibodies bind most efficiently at temperatures below 37 C; some will not bind at all at 37 C and react best at 0–4 C. It is now believed that this temperature-mediated effect reflects a structural change in the red cell membrane that enhances the antibody-antigen reaction at low temperature. Most cold-reactive antibodies are IgM, usually with anti-I or -i activity. Cold antibodies of the IgG class are found in the syndrome, paroxysmal cold hemoglobinuria, which is a complication of syphilis and certain viral infections. In cold weather, for example, cold antibodies bind to red cell antigens in the distal extremities and initiate the early stages of complement fixation. As the blood warms during its passage through the central circulation, the Ig is released, but complement components remain bound and, if present at high enough concentration, render the cell liable to macrophage-mediated hemolysis. When complement fixation is sufficiently vigorous, direct intravascular hemolysis may be triggered. Warm-reactive antibodies bind to red cells most effectively at 37 C. Both IgG and IgM of this type are recognized.

6.4.4 ANTIBODY-MEDIATED AGGLUTINATION REACTIONS

Ig are often distinguished as "complete" or "incomplete" antibodies depending upon their agglutinating properties in vitro. "Complete" or "saline" antibodies will agglutinate the appropriately antigenic red cells in isotonic NaCl. They usually are IgM. "Incomplete" antibodies, regularly IgG, require special tests in order to demonstrate the interaction of antibody and red cell, since the antibody alone will not agglutinate red cells. Red cells are normally maintained in their dispersed suspension by a net negative charge on the cell membrane due principally to sialic acid residues. Antibodies, to effect agglutination, must overcome this ionic repulsive force (called the zeta potential), which keeps adjacent red cells at least 30 nm apart. The two antigen-binding sites of IgG span less than 30 nm, and IgG usually cannot agglutinate red cells. IgM, a pentamer Ig, can span up to 50 nm between binding sites and can more easily bridge adjacent red cells. When the density of red cell antigenic sites is extremely high, this distinction may disappear. For example, whereas IgG anti-Rh cannot agglutinate Rh-positive red cells (the maximum number of D sites is only about 30,000/red cell), the IgG variety of anti-A is an effective agglutinin (A antigen is represented by up to 1,000,000 antigenic sites in adult A_1 red cells).

The presence of bound "incomplete" antibodies can be demonstrated by any of several technics, which either: (1) promote agglutination by decreasing the red cell-repulsive negative charges (i.e., increase the dielectric properties of the medium by performing the reaction in albumin or decrease the red cell charge itself with sialidase or protease treatment), or (2) agglutinate IgG-sensitized red cells by means of antibodies to human IgG produced in another species. The latter approach forms the principle of the clinically invaluable Coombs test used for detection of nonagglutinating anti-red cell antibodies, for detection of autoimmune red cell antibodies and for determining the titer of maternal red cell antibodies during pregnancies with blood group incompatibility (hemolytic disease of the newborn; see section 6.9).

The antiglobulin (or Coombs) test, used to detect "incomplete" antibodies, may be em-

ployed in two ways. The *direct antiglobulin test* detects the presence of Ig or complement components on the patient's own red cells. The patient's cells are reacted with an antiglobulin antiserum and scored for agglutination. The specificity of the test depends on the specificities of the antiglobulin; a broad-spectrum reagent will detect both Ig and complement. Highly specialized antibodies may be prepared against individual Ig types, if necessary.

The *indirect antiglobulin test* detects "incomplete" red cell antibodies in the serum. Normal red cells are incubated with the patient's serum, washed thoroughly and tested for agglutination with appropriate antiglobulin antiserum, just as in the direct test.

6.5 Role of Complement

As already noted, complement components participate in hemolysis of red cells by at least two independent mechanisms: (1) promoting adherence of sensitized cells to macrophages of the reticuloendothelial system, which results in erythrophagocytosis; and (2) activation of the complete lytic complement system and generation of a lesion in the red cell membrane, which permits osmotic hemolysis of the sensitized cell. The following steps provide an outline of the process of complement-mediated red cell injury (Fig. 6–5):

Fig. 6–5.—Simplified schema of the complement reactions that can result in red cell sequestration and phagocytosis or in direct intravascular hemolysis.

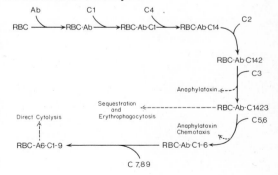

1. The immunologically specific adherence of antibody with complement-fixing activity to red cell antigens provides receptor sites for attachment of the first complement component, C1. This reaction requires two Fc complement receptor sites within 25–40 nm of each other. Thus, a single pentameric IgM molecule bound to the red cell membrane may initiate complement fixation. However, over 2,000 IgG may be needed to ensure that at least one close doublet will be formed. Furthermore, the distribution of antigenic sites is critical. The sparsely distributed Rh antigens are far apart, so that red cells sensitized with an IgG anti-Rh do not bind complement, no matter how much antibody is bound.

2. Binding of C1 initiates esterolytic activity in a portion of C1, which effects the binding of several molecules of C4 and C2. The C42 complex has enzymatic activity, which, in turn,

3. Cleaves a fragment from C3 and promotes the binding of hundreds of molecules of C3 to the red cell surface. C3 has two biologically active portions. One site is recognized by macrophages and mediates adherence to and phagocytosis by the reticuloendothelial system. The other site has proteolytic activity, which promotes the fixation of C5. Both of these biologic properties are subject to rapid inactivation by a serum enzyme, C3b inactivator.

4. C5 binding and the subsequent sequential attachment of C6, C7, C8 and C9 establish the membrane lesion that increases ionic permeability and causes intravascular osmotic lysis. The human complement system is not particularly efficient in C5 fixation. This may explain why so many red cell immune reactions result in C3 binding and hemolysis by red cell sequestration in the reticuloendothelial system rather than intravascular hemolysis. When complement fixation is vigorous and complete, as in the case of mismatched transfusion with ABO-incompatible blood, there are generated considerable amounts of complement cleavage products, some of which (C3a and C5a) have potent anaphylatoxic properties. The anaphylactoid reactions observed during severe transfusion reactions may be due to these products.

6.6 Role of Reticuloendothelial System

Participation of one or both of the two major reticuloendothelial organs, spleen and liver, is pivotal to the pathophysiology of most instances of immune hemolytic disease. These two organs provide the body with mechanisms for the elimination of red cells, with a wide variety of types and degrees of injury. In this respect the liver and spleen are remarkably complementary.

The liver receives a vast blood supply through its relatively simple sinusoidal vasculature lined with Kupffer cells and other potential macrophages. The liver is capable of rapid sequestration of severely injured red cells including, for example, cells sensitized by complement-binding IgM antibodies.

The spleen, although it receives less than 5% of the cardiac output, exercises an extraordinary sensitivity for sequestering and destroying minimally injured erythrocytes, including cells sensitized by IgG, whether complement fixing or not. Unlike the liver, the splenic reticuloendothelial system is disposed in a complex filterlike arrangement (the Billroth cords) that forces circulating red cells to pass small fenestrations in close contact with tissue macrophages (Fig. 6–6). Cells that have lost their natural pliability or that are abnormally adherent to macrophages are retarded in their passage through the spleen. The splenic environment, which features hypoxia, hypoglycemia and acidosis among its characteristics, imposes a severe metabolic burden on red cells trapped or slowed in this manner. The combination of metabolic and immunologic injuries ultimately results in permanent splenic sequestration and erythrophagocytosis.

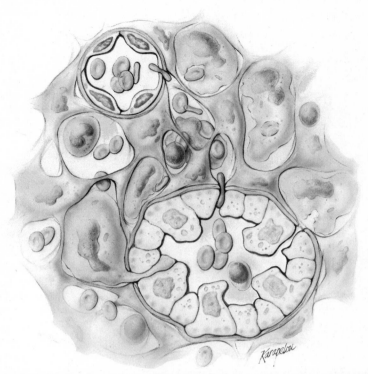

Fig. 6–6.—The splenic red pulp, site of erythrocyte sequestration and phagocytosis. Red cells enter the Billroth cord from a terminal arteriole or capillary *(top left)*, percolate through the fine spaces formed by reticular fibers and macrophages, then exit by gaining access to a splenic sinusoid *(bottom right)* through small fenestrations in the sinusoidal basement membrane. Injured red cells are retarded in passage and may be recognized by macrophages for erythrophagocytosis. Bound immunoglobulin or complement provides one such signal to the macrophages.

6.7 Autoimmune Hemolytic Anemias (AIHA)

These disorders comprise that group of hemolytic anemias in which shortened red cell life span is mediated by components of the immune system, with specificity directed at the patient's own red cells. For convenience, we shall also consider paroxysmal nocturnal hemoglobinuria (section 6.8) and hemolytic disease of the newborn (section 6.9), although they are not strictly autoimmune diseases. Major clinical patterns can be recognized among the AIHA, and these correlate reasonably well with properties of the specific autoantibodies and of the implicated red cell antigens. A useful classification is provided in Table 6–1, and an outline

TABLE 6–1.—CLASSIFICATION OF ACQUIRED IMMUNE HEMOLYTIC DISORDERS

With warm-reactive autoantibodies
  Idiopathic
  Secondary
    Associated with lymphoreticular malignancies, SLE, infections, ovarian teratoma, infectious mononucleosis
With cold-reactive autoantibodies
  Idiopathic (cold agglutinin disease)
  Secondary
    Associated with *Mycoplasma pneumoniae*, infectious mononucleosis, lymphomas
  Paroxysmal cold hemoglobinuria
    Associated with viral infections or syphilis
Drug-related
  Haptene mechanism ("penicillin")
  Immune complex ("innocent bystander") mechanism (quinidine, quinine, stibophen)
  True autoimmune anti-red cell antibodies (α-methyl dopa)

TABLE 6–2.—PROPERTIES OF AUTOANTIBODIES IN
AUTOIMMUNE HEMOLYTIC ANEMIA

ANTIBODY CHARACTERISTICS	IMMUNO-GLOBULIN CLASS	ANTIBODIES DETECTED BY DIRECT ANTIGLOBULIN TEST	ANTIBODY SPECIFICITY
Warm-reactive	IgG	IgG	Frequently "Rh-related"
Warm-reactive	IgG	IgG + complement	Undefined
Warm-reactive	IgG	Complement alone	Undefined
Cold-reactive	IgM	Complement alone	Anti-I, -i; other
Cold-reactive (Donath-Landsteiner)	IgG	Complement alone	Anti-P

of some salient properties of the usual red cell autoantibodies will be found in Table 6–2. The major clinical features of the principal syndromes are listed in Table 6–3.

6.7.1 AIHA with Warm-Type (IgG) Autoantibodies

This may be found at all ages; the higher incidence among older age groups is probably related to a strong association with the lymphoproliferative disorders. Indeed, secondary warm-type AIHA, associated principally with lymphoid disease and systemic lupus erythematosus (SLE), accounts for about 50% of the incidence of this hemolytic syndrome. The incidence of positive direct antiglobulin tests probably exceeds the incidence of clinically overt warm-type hemolysis by several fold, attesting to the wide variability in severity of this syndrome. When clinically apparent, the disease varies from mild chronic hemolysis, readily compensated by marrow erythroid hyperplasia, to fulminating hemolysis, with prostration, jaundice and profound anemia. The clinical severity of the hemolytic anemia does not correlate well with the intensity of the direct antiglob-

TABLE 6–3.—CLINICAL FEATURES OF AUTOIMMUNE HEMOLYTIC ANEMIAS

CLINICAL FEATURES	WARM-TYPE AUTOIMMUNE	COLD AGGLUTININ SYNDROME	PAROXYSMAL COLD HEMOGLOBINURIA
Age at onset	Childhood to old age	Usually older age (except postinfectious type)	Often young adult
Severity of anemia	Variable	Usually moderate or mild	Acute and intermittent forms may be severe
Hemoglobinuria	Rare	Present in severe cases only	Usual
Other symptoms	Rare	Cold intolerance	Rigor, anaphylatoxic symptoms
Splenomegaly	Frequent	Usual	Intermittent
Vascular phenomena on exposure to cold	None	Raynaud's phenomenon	Cold urticaria, paresthesias
Benefit from			
Adrenocortical steroids	Usual	No value at tolerable levels	Not yet defined
Splenectomy	Frequent	No value	Not yet defined
Immuno-suppressive therapy	May be effective	May be effective	Not yet defined
Cold avoidance	None	Effective	Effective

ulin test. The following rough guidelines may be drawn:

1. Intravascular hemolysis due to warm-type autoantibodies requires a high titer of efficient complement-binding antibody and a high density of antigenic sites sufficient to achieve full complement activation. This combination of factors is relatively rare.

2. IgG-sensitized red cells will be preferentially destroyed in the spleen where immune adherence and spherocytosis lead to highly efficient sequestration.

3. Red cells sensitized with both IgG and the C3 component of complement can be sequestered by both spleen and liver. Whereas the liver reticuloendothelial system displays an almost absolute requirement for complement in order to effect red cell sequestration, the spleen is less stringent.

6.7.2 TREATMENT OF WARM-TYPE AIHA

Adrenocortical steroids are the first line of therapeutics in warm-type disease and are effective, at least temporarily, in up to 80–90% of patients with the idiopathic form. Recent experimental studies strongly suggest that a major effect of the steroid hormones is to decrease the efficiency of the reticuloendothelial system in sequestering immunologically injured red cells, perhaps by decreasing the affinity of macrophages for IgG and complement sites on the sensitized red cells. Steroids probably also have some immunosuppressive activity; serum anti-red cell antibody titers may fall slowly while steroids are given; and the direct antiglobulin test may, but need not, become weaker or negative.

If steroid therapy at clinically tolerable doses fails to control hemolysis, splenectomy is considered, especially if major splenic sequestration and minimal hepatic sequestration can be demonstrated by ^{51}Cr labeling technics (see section 2.3.1). If splenectomy fails or is inappropriate, a course of immuno-

suppressive therapy, e.g., azathioprine, may be tried.

6.7.3 COLD-REACTIVE AUTOANTIBODIES

These are usually IgM, although cold-reactive IgG syndromes are described. Cold-reactive IgM is a complement-fixing agglutinin and produces morbidity by three mechanisms:

1. It agglutinates red cells in the distal vasculature at low ambient temperatures. This produces stasis, cyanosis and Raynaud-like reactions. At the same time the autoantibody promotes attachment of the initial components of complement, up to C3. As the blood reaches the warm central circulation, the IgM is released and the agglutinates disperse, but C3 remains cell bound.

2. If the IgM is a vigorous complement-binding antibody and the number of cell-bound C3 molecules is high enough, then C5–C9 are attached, and brisk intravascular hemolysis is precipitated. This is relatively rare in clinical experience.

3. Alternatively, C3-sensitized red cells are sequestered by the reticuloendothelial system, particularly in the liver. If the degree of C3 fixation is low, sequestration may be transient. It is speculated that under these conditions bound C3 is destroyed or inactivated by the serum enzyme, C3b inactivator, before phagocytosis can occur. If the red cells are more heavily coated with C3, permanent sequestration, erythrophagocytosis and hemolysis result.

These clinical patterns are typical of idiopathic *chronic cold agglutinin disease* as well as the secondary cold agglutinin syndromes associated with Mycoplasma infection, infectious mononucleosis and lymphoproliferative disorders (see section 12.1.2). In most instances the IgM autoantibody has anti-I specificity. The autoantibody that appears during infectious mononucleosis is anti-i. Since most adults' red cells are poorly reactive with anti-i (they have predominantly I antigenicity; see section 6.3.3), clinical hemolysis is very rare (0.1% or less) in infectious mononucleosis.

The cold agglutinin syndromes due to infections are generally acute and self-limited and, although they may be severe, they respond to supportive care including warmth, rest and, when needed, transfusion. The lymphomas require treatment according to their type and distribution. Idiopathic chronic cold agglutinin disease usually is unresponsive to tolerable doses of steroid hormones, and splenectomy is predictably of little help. Alkylating agents, e.g., chlorambucil, may be distinctly beneficial in some instances of the disease.

The cold-reactive autoantibodies in *paroxysmal cold hemoglobinuria,* unlike the other cold hemolytic syndromes, are complement-fixing IgG, almost always displaying antibody activity against a very common blood group antigen called P. The chronic, episodic form of the disease is one of the protean but rare manifestations of syphilis. An acute, fulminating but self-limited variant is seen 7–14 days following various viral infections including chickenpox and measles. Hemoglobinuria, back pain and cramps, vasomotor reactions and anaphylactoid reactions are attributed to complement-mediated intravascular hemolysis. In both syndromes vigorous supportive measures generally suffice. The postviral syndrome is nonrecurrent and even the chronic syphilitic syndrome is clinically relatively benign.

6.7.4 DRUG-INDUCED AUTOIMMUNE HEMOLYSIS

Antibody-mediated hemolysis is associated with exposure to certain drugs. At least three different hemolytic mechanisms have been described.

1. *Haptene mechanism.* Patients receiving prolonged very high doses of penicillin (e.g., in treatment of subacute bacterial endocarditis) not uncommonly form IgG anti-penicillin antibodies that can react with penicillin bound to the patient's own red cells. These IgG antibodies are much more common than are actual instances of hemolysis, and those anemias observed vary from mild to severe. IgM antipenicillin antibodies are quite common in treated patients but do not participate in this hemolytic process.

2. The *"innocent bystander" mechanism.* Certain IgM antibodies against drugs including stilbophen, quinine, quinidine, α-aminobenzoic acid, sulfonamides and phenacetin react with the drug in the serum, forming antigen-antibody complexes, which are then adsorbed to red cell membranes where they promote complement fixation and hemolysis.

3. *True drug-induced AIHA.* A high percentage (10–20%) of patients receiving α-methyldopa for protracted periods develop a positive direct antiglobulin test. A much smaller fraction develop overt hemolysis of the warm-reactive IgG variety, exhibiting Rh specificity. The drug itself is not directly responsible for the positive Coombs test since the antibody lacks any anti-drug activity. Withdrawal of α-methyldopa leads to gradual decrease in the strength of the Coombs test and amelioration of the anemia, if there was overt hemolysis. The mechanism whereby the drug initiates an autoimmune reaction is unknown.

6.8 Paroxysmal Nocturnal Hemoglobinuria (PNH)

Hemolytic anemia mediated by components of the complement system but without participation of specific (antibody) immune mechanisms is characteristic of the acquired disorder, PNH. Despite its name this disease appears to affect all three cellular elements and may be the result of some as yet undetected acquired injury at the level of the hematopoietic stem cell. Pancytopenia is common but the pathognomonic feature is the presence of a population of red cells exquisitely sensitive to the hemolytic action of complement. Complement activation in this condition bypasses the requirement for antibody and the antibody-dependent fixation of C1, C2 and C4. PNH red cells are significantly more efficient in completing the sequential addition of C3 and C5–C9 than are normal cells, whether mediated by the bypass mechanism or by antibody. The diagnosis should be suspected (1) if there is a history of anemia and dark urine on awakening (nocturnal hemoglobinuria), and (2) in virtually any instance of pancytopenia not readily explained by other mechanisms. A high incidence of thromboembolic disease also may accompany PNH, perhaps due to thromboplastic substances released during intravascular hemolysis, and should also raise suspicion of this diagnosis. Aplastic anemia may occur in relation to PNH, and acute leukemia occasionally occurs as a sequel to the disorder.

Lysis of PNH cells can be triggered in vitro by (1) lowering the ionic strength of the medium without changing its osmotic properties by adding a solution of sucrose ("sugar-water" test), or (2) incubation with fresh acidified normal serum (Ham test). In either case, complement lysis is initiated in PNH but not in normal cells, and the diagnosis is based on one of these two tests.

6.9 Hemolytic Disease of the Newborn (Erythroblastosis Fetalis)

This condition arises when maternal IgG specific for the fetus' red cell antigens is transported across the placenta into the fetal circulation and initiates hemolysis by the fetal reticuloendothelial system. The involved antigens are almost always either from the Rh or ABO system. Clinical manifestations range from mild to catastrophic, including intrauterine fetal death (hydrops fetalis), profound postnatal hemolytic anemia and severe postnatal jaundice with neurologic damage due to hyperbilirubinemia (kernicterus). The pathogenesis is now reasonably well established and it is possible to avoid or prevent the disorder in many instances by measures designed to prevent maternal immunization to fetal erythrocyte antigens.

6.9.1 FETAL-MATERNAL ABO-INCOMPATIBILITY

Although ABO-incompatibility occurs in 20–25% of pregnancies, the incidence of hemolytic disease of the newborn due to ABO sensitization is low (less than 0.5%) and hydrops fetalis is virtually unknown. The reason for this stems from what we already know about the ABO system (see section 6.3.1). Only IgG will cross the placenta; significant titers of IgG anti-A and anti-B are confined to type O mothers. Further, the A and B antigens are not fully developed in the fetus and infant. Lastly, and perhaps most significant, A and B antigens are not confined to red cells; maternal antibody reaching the fetal tissues may be neutralized by a large pool of nonerythrocytic antigen. Treatment is rarely necessary in ABO-incompatibility. If postnatal bilirubin levels rise to dangerous levels, a single exchange transfusion usually will suffice until the hemolysis subsides and the infant liver itself is competent to clear the blood of bilirubin.

6.9.2 RH-INCOMPATIBILITY

The D antigen is the most immunogenic of the Rh antigens, and most instances of Rh hemolytic disease of the newborn are due to the presence of a D (D/D or D/d) embryo in an Rh-negative (d/d) mother. Until the recent introduction of prophylactic measures to prevent maternal sensitization, the incidence of Rh disease was between 0.5% and 0.75% of births. Unlike ABO disease, Rh-incompatibility can produce severe morbidity ranging from hydrops fetalis to kernicterus.

Rh-negative mothers do not have natural anti-Rh antibodies; they must be stimulated by mismatched transfusion or by the small but significant infusion of fetal cells (1–5 ml) that reach the maternal circulation during the third stage of labor. These fetal cells can initiate Rh-sensitivity, which will be manifested during a subsequent Rh-positive pregnancy when maternal anti-Rh IgG is transported across the placenta to the fetus and causes hemolysis. It is known, however, that, if mother and fetus are both ABO-incompatible *and* Rh-incompatible, then Rh-immunization is much *less* likely to occur. It is speculated that the fetus' Rh-positive red cells are rapidly destroyed in the mother's circulation by her natural anti-A or anti-B and rendered ineffective as immunogens. The presently available highly effective method of protecting Rh-negative mothers from immunization by fetal cells may actually be a variant of this natural mechanism.

6.9.3 PREVENTION OF MATERNAL SENSITIZATION

It has been conclusively shown that if Rh-negative mothers with Rh-positive husbands are given an injection of human anti-Rh antiserum at the time of delivery of their first and all subsequent pregnancies, the unavoidable infusion with fetal red cells that occurs at delivery will fail to excite an immune reaction. This prophylaxis does not protect against an anamnestic response in an already immunized mother.

6.9.4 MANAGEMENT OF FETO-MATERNAL INCOMPATIBILITY

Maternal anti-Rh titers must be followed during all pregnancies in Rh-negative women carrying a potentially Rh-positive fetus. If maternal titers rise, it is necessary to monitor the fetal response by examination of the amniotic fluid for bilirubin content. If fetal bilirubin levels rise early in pregnancy (before 24 weeks), hydrops is likely. Small transfusions of Rh-negative (type O) blood administered in this situation into the fetal peritoneum by transuterine injection may suppress fetal production of Rh-positive cells and permit pregnancy to continue until

it is safe to undertake cesarean section and to continue with exchange transfusions until the infant can handle his own bilirubin production. Some neonates from Rh-incompatible pregnancies are born looking normal but proceed to develop dangerously elevated bilirubin levels shortly after delivery. Repeated exchange transfusions are required to tide these infants past the threat of kernicteric brain damage.

6.10 Hereditary Spherocytic Anemia (HSA)

HSA is a rare familial disorder inherited with the pattern of autosomal dominance, characterized by hemolytic anemia, microspherocytes in the peripheral blood, splenomegaly and invariable response to splenectomy. The primary red cell lesion appears to be in the red cell membrane, but accelerated hemolysis is absolutely dependent upon the unique structural and metabolic features of the Billroth cords of the spleen (see section 6.6).

The clinical severity of the disorder varies considerably, although severe anemia is most unusual, except transiently when acute infections, brief hypoplastic episodes or folate deficiency may intervene. Red cell life span is shortened, but this is generally well compensated by erythroid hyperplasia in the marrow. Accelerated red cell turnover nevertheless results in an elevated unconjugated serum bilirubin level (rarely higher than 3 – 4 mg%) which, because it is sustained, predisposes to pigmentary gallstones, cholecystitis, cholangitis and biliary obstruction. Splenomegaly is almost invariable and is thought to be due to chronically overactive sequestration of red cells.

6.10.1 DIAGNOSTIC FEATURES

The peripheral blood shows reticulocytosis and the presence of microspherocytes in variable, often small numbers. These sphero-

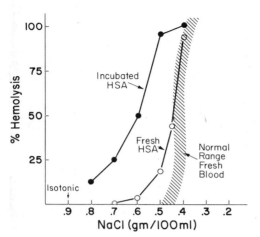

Fig. 6–7.—Osmotic fragility curves for normal blood, for fresh hereditary spherocytosis (HSA) blood and for HSA blood after 24 hours of sterile incubation. The increased sensitivity of HSA blood to hemolysis (hemolysis starts at a concentration of NaCl nearer to isotonic) is accentuated by incubation.

cytes are a consequence of the loss of small fragments of red cell membranes and a decreased surface/volume ratio. The spherocytes are more sensitive to osmotic hemolysis than are normal red cells. This is the basis of the *osmotic fragility test* in which red cells are suspended in a series of saline solutions of decreasing concentration (Fig. 6–7). Normal red cells swell and lyse relatively abruptly between 0.35% and 0.5% NaCl (isotonic NaCl is 0.9%). Red cells of HSA show a moderately increased osmotic fragility plus a small population of highly fragile red cells that may begin to hemolyze at 0.7% NaCl. These sensitive cells are spherocytes that have been severely injured metabolically ("conditioned") by prolonged sojourn

within the spleen's inhospitable environment. No portion of the reticuloendothelial system other than the spleen appears capable of accelerated sequestration of HSA red cells, and so splenectomy is inevitably successful in alleviating hemolysis, anemia and the biliary complications.

6.10.2 NATURE OF RED CELL DEFECT IN HSA

The following elements comprise a summary of the present understanding of this inherited lesion that is intrinsic to the red cell:

1. *An abnormally high rate of Na+ flux into HSA red cells.* This does not itself appear to be the primary spherocyte-producing lesion, since erythrophagocytosis, not osmotic hemolysis, is the mechanism of red cell destruction in vivo.

2. *Rate of red cell glycolysis slightly increased over normal.* This appears to be due to the metabolic requirements of the Na+–K+ membrane pump needed to maintain osmotic equilibrium. When red cells are incubated sterilely in the absence of glucose, HSA cells show much more severe deterioration in osmotic fragility than do normal red cells. This is the basis of the incubated osmotic fragility test (see Fig. 6–7), which may be used to demonstrate the HSA defect when the standard osmotic fragility test is equivocal.

3. *Hypothesis:* The mutant HSA gene may determine a structural abnormality of the red cell membrane. This abnormality may be responsible for the accelerated ion flux as well as for rigidity, fragmentation and spherocyte formation.

7

Hemolytic Anemia: Defects of Red Cell Metabolism

7.1 Normal Red Cell Energy Metabolism

THE ENERGY NEEDS of mature erythrocytes are met exclusively by glucose metabolism. Mitochondria, cytochromes and enzymes of the Krebs (tricarboxylic, aerobic) cycle are absent from erythrocytes. Red cell glucose may be catabolized either by "anaerobic glycolysis" (Embden-Meyerhof pathway) to pyruvate and lactate or by the pentose phosphate pathway (hexose monophosphate shunt), which generates CO_2 directly and by the triose reactions contributes to pyruvate and lactate production (Fig. 7–1).

Normally, red cell energy requirements are small but critical. These basic energy needs include the following:

1. *Ion pump mechanisms* necessary to maintain osmotic stability. This transport function is driven by adenosine triphosphate (ATP), generated largely by the membrane-bound enzyme, phosphoglycerate kinase, which catalyzes the conversion of 1,3-diphosphoglycerate to 3-diphosphoglycerate.

2. The *methemoglobin-reduction system,* which maintains hemoglobin in its function Fe^{++} form by reducing Fe^{+++}–hemoglobin (methemoglobin). This enzyme system (methemoglobin reductase, or diaphorase as it is also called), is driven by reduced nicotinamide adenine dinucleotide (NADH), generated from nicotinamide adenine dinucleotide (NAD) by the enzyme glyceraldehyde-3-phosphate dehydrogenase.

3. The *glutathione reductase system,* integral to the protection of critical sulfhydryl groups in hemoglobin and of other proteins essential for red cell function and integrity. This system is dependent upon reduced nicotinamide adenine dinucleotide phosphate (NADPH) generated from NADP exclusively by the pentose phosphate pathway and its two principal enzymes, glucose-6-phosphate dehydrogenase (G-6-PD) and phosphogluconate dehydrogenase.

4. *Synthesis of NAD* from nicotinic acid,

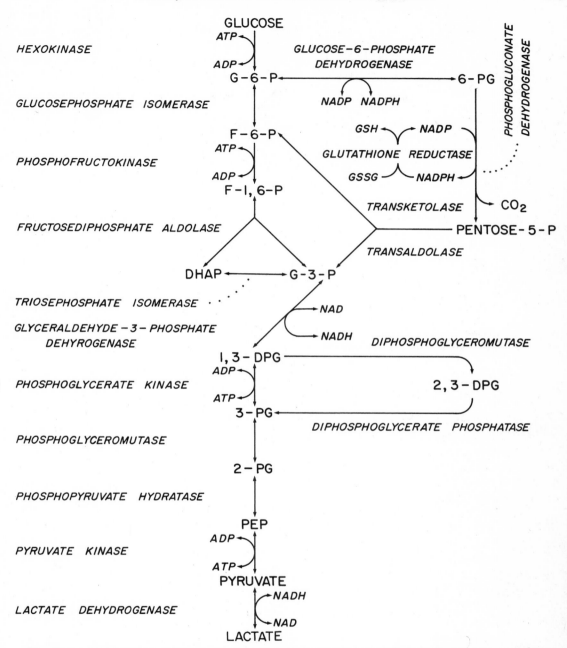

Fig. 7–1.—Intermediary glucose metabolism in the red cell. 6-G-P = glucose-6-phosphate; F-6-P = fructose-6-phosphate; F-1, 6-P = fructose 1, 6-diphosphate; DHAP = dihydroxyacetone-phosphate; G-3-P = glyceraldehyde-3-phosphate; 1,3-DPG = 1,3-diphosphoglycerate; 3-PG = 3-phosphoglycerate; 2-PG = 2-phosphoglycerate; PEP = 2-phosphoenolpyruvate; 6-PG = 6-phosphogluconate.

glutamine, glucose and inorganic phosphate. NADP is formed by the reaction of NAD with ATP.

As erythrocytes mature in the circulation, there is a decrease in activity of a number of enzymes including hexokinase, phosphohexose isomerase, phosphofructokinase, aldolase, triosephosphate isomerase, glyceraldehyde phosphate dehydrogenase, G-6-PD and others. These decreases in enzyme activity are associated with other changes in the erythrocyte as it ages in the circulation, such as an increased concentration of methemoglobin, decreased concentration of K^+ and increased concentration of Na^+, increased susceptibility to immune hemolysis, increased mechanical fragility and increased susceptibility to intracellular denaturation of hemoglobin and stromal proteins by oxidants.

7.2 Inherited Disorders of Energy Metabolism

Functionally abnormal mutants of many of the enzymes of the Embden-Meyerhof and pentose phosphate pathways are known. Of these, deficient G-6-PD activity constitutes over 95% of the clinically important inherited metabolic defects of the erythrocyte and, indeed, is the most frequent of all clinically apparent hereditary enzyme deficiencies world-wide. The next most common, albeit rare, red cell enzyme disorder is pyruvate kinase (PK) deficiency. Both of these will be considered, illustrating as they do the hematologic consequences of metabolic defects in both the Embden-Meyerhof and pentose phosphate pathways.

7.3 G-6-PD Deficiency and Pentose Phosphate Pathway

Activity of the pentose phosphate pathway, which normally accounts for a minor fraction of glucose metabolism in the RBC, is affected by the redox state of the red cell and, in particular, by the demand for reduced glutathione (glutathione-SH). This molecule, as already noted, is required for reduction or protection of sulfhydryl groups in critical regions of essential cellular proteins that are subject to oxidative denaturation. The activity of the first enzyme in the hexose monophosphate (HMP) pathway, G-6-PD, is modulated by the intracellular concentrations of NADP and NADPH, being stimulated by NADP and inhibited by NADPH. When red cells are exposed to a variety of agents, including potentially oxidative drugs and as yet unknown products of bacterial and viral infections, inflammation and other metabolic disturbances (e.g., diabetic ketoacidosis), the demand for glutathione-SH increases and is met by accelerated production of NADPH from NADP in the pentose phosphate pathway. The NADPH generated is available as a hydrogen donor for the glutathione reductase reaction.

In the presence of genetically determined deficiency of G-6-PD activity, the pentose phosphate pathway and the generation of NADPH cannot respond adequately to meet metabolic demands. Consequently, oxidative denaturation of critical proteins occurs, especially hemoglobin, resulting in gross alterations in red cell structure and physical properties. Oxidation of hemoglobin leads to precipitation of the denatured protein in insoluble masses called Heinz bodies, which can be visualized with supravital stains or by electron microscopy. These rigid intracellular precipitates, perhaps coupled with other critical injuries, result in an inflexible red cell unable to negotiate the splenic and hepatic sinusoids (see section 6.6). Sequestration by the reticuloendothelial system and hemolysis by erythrophagocytosis constitute the usual outcome. If the injury is extreme, intravascular hemolysis can be prominent, even fulminating.

7.3.1 GENETIC VARIANTS

Over 80 allelic variants of G-6-PD are known. The G-6-PD locus is X-linked;

males are hemizygous and fully express the biologic activity of the allele they carry. Heterozygous females are mosaic, due to random X-inactivation according to the Lyon hypothesis. Clinical expression of alleles for defective enzyme activity in a female will depend upon the statistical incidence of one or the other active X chromosome in her erythroid cell population. The usual alleles, with normal enzymatic activity, are designated G-6-PD^A, common among black African populations, and G-6-PD^B, the gene for the common isoenzyme in other populations. It is assumed, but not yet proved, that most of the variants differ by single amino acid substitutions, in a manner analogous to mutant hemoglobins (see section 8.3). About half of the known variants are detected only by virtue of differences in electrophoretic mobility or by other physical properties; their enzymatic activity is normal or so close to normal as to produce no clinical manifestations.

Another group of variants has deficient enzyme activity that predisposes to hemolytic anemia but only when the patient is exposed to oxidant drugs, infections or metabolic disorders such as diabetic ketoacidosis. The A$^-$ variant, common in black populations, is of this sort. G-6-PD^{Mediterranean} represents a similar but even more severe deficiency, with a high incidence among populations from the Mediterranean littoral, e.g., Greeks, Sardinians, Italians, Sephardic Jews and Kurds.

A third, far more rare group of alleles found predominantly in West European populations results in a chronic hemolytic anemia that does not depend upon exogenous oxidative stress. The enzymatic activity of these variants appears to be inadequate to protect red cells even from normal wear and tear. Overall, the high frequency of deleterious G-6-PD genes provides an example of genetic polymorphism. It is proposed that mutant G-6-PD alleles confer protection from *Plasmodium falciparum* in malaria-endemic populations.

7.3.2 PATHOPHYSIOLOGY OF G-6-PD DEFICIENCY

The hemolytic severity of G-6-PD deficiency is a complex function of several factors, including:

1. *Age of RBC.* G-6-PD activity, even in genetically normal red cells, deteriorates progressively as the cell ages. Reticulocytes and young erythrocytes have higher enzyme activity than do older cells. Older red cells are more sensitive to oxidative denaturation, especially if enzyme activity is genetically deficient.

2. Dose or *concentration of oxidant drug* or metabolite.

3. *G-6-PD allele carried.* G-6-PD^{A-} is of moderate severity. Reticulocytes and young erythrocytes are relatively resistant to hemolysis, and the degree of hemolysis will depend largely on the dose of oxidant administered. Initially, hemolysis will be brisk while all red cells with less than critical levels of G-6-PD are being hemolyzed. Continued administration of drug at the same dosage produces an equilibrium between accelerated erythropoiesis and hemolysis. An increased dose will produce another acceleration of hemolysis until a new equilibrium is achieved. G-6-PD^{Mediterranean}, on the other hand, is a more severe deficiency. There may be no equilibrium phase, and anemia may be progressive until the offending drug is withdrawn.

Favism is a peculiar manifestation found in a small proportion of individuals carrying G-6-PD^{Mediterranean}. Eating the fava bean, or even inhaling fava pollen, may precipitate a fulminating hemolytic crisis, with massive intravascular hemolysis. The nature of interaction between a fava component and G-6-PD-deficient red cells is not known.

7.3.3 DIAGNOSIS

G-6-PD deficiency may be suspected on the basis of the historical relation between

TABLE 7–1.—HEMOLYTIC AGENTS
IN G-6-PD DEFICIENCY

DRUGS
   Sulfonamides and related compounds
   Sulfones
   Naphthalene
   Methylene blue
   Acetylsalicylic acid
   Nitrofurantoin
   Furazolidone
   Primaquine-type drugs
   Vitamins K and K_1
   Quinine and Quinidine
   Antipyrene
   Probenecid
   Acetanilide
   Phenylhydrazine
   Acetophenetidin
   Chloroquine
   Chloramphenicol
OTHER FACTORS
   Fava bean and pollen
   Infections: respiratory viruses, hepatitis, infectious
      mononucleosis, bacterial pneumonia, septicemia
   Diabetic ketoacidosis
   Uremia

drug and hemolytic anemia. It is confirmed by assays of G-6-PD activity. In the presence of an elevated reticulocyte count, only a low G-6-PD level is meaningful; a normal level must be confirmed by a repeat assay at a later time when the proportion of young erythrocytes has returned to normal levels. The mosaic distribution of normal and deficient red cells in a heterozygous female may only be revealed by a cytologic test of G-6-PD activity, which distinguishes the subpopulation of deficient cells by means of redox-sensitive dyes such as the tetrazolium reagents.

Table 7–1 provides a partial list of agents or factors that have been shown to be capable of precipitating hemolysis in G-6-PD-deficient subjects.

7.4 PK Deficiency and Embden-Meyerhof Pathway

This relatively rare autosomal recessive deficiency produces hemolytic anemia only when present in the homozygous state. The enzyme catalyzes the formation of pyruvate from phosphoenolpyruvate with the generation of one mole of ATP. Deficiency of the enzyme seriously compromises glycolysis, alters the concentration of glycolytic intermediary metabolites and decreases ATP production. Reticulocytes, which have residual ATP-generating activity in the Krebs cycle, suffer less severely from PK deficiency than do more mature erythrocytes.

Affected individuals often manifest anemia and jaundice early in infancy or childhood; indeed, severe neonatal jaundice and kernicterus are reported, and exchange transfusion may be required. Biliary complications are not uncommon, due to bilirubin stones. Moderate splenomegaly is usual and splenectomy frequently is accompanied by amelioration of the transfusion requirement. The precise diagnosis requires enzyme assay as there are no other pathognomonic features. It should be emphasized that in all hemolytic anemias in which an enzyme deficiency is suspected, diagnosis depends upon specific assays for the level of enzyme activity in hemolysates prepared from the patient's RBC.

Properties of Hemoglobin: Defects in Hemoglobin and Hemoglobin Synthesis

8.1 Introduction

THE HEMOGLOBINOPATHIES are caused by genetically determined lesions that alter the structure or quantity of hemoglobin produced in differentiating erythroid cells. The clinical syndromes that result from these genetic lesions depend upon the nature of the mutation. Broadly, mutations may affect the structure of the polypeptide chains of hemoglobin (the hemoglobin variants or hemoglobinopathies proper) or the mechanisms that govern the rate and amount of globin polypeptide chains produced (thalassemia syndromes). These two categories of genetic defects are not mutually exclusive. Structural abnormalities (hemoglobin variants) are now known that are associated with biochemical and clinical manifestations typical of regulatory mutants (the thalassemias). Structural mutations display a variety of manifestations, depending upon which site in

63

the molecule is altered. As might be predicted, most point mutations (single amino acid substitutions due to a single nucleotide base alteration) lead to no biochemical or clinical effect whatsoever, since many single amino acids may be changed without altering function or physical properties of the hemoglobin molecule. There are, however, a number of extremely critical regions in the molecule, and substitutions in these regions may be pathogenic.

8.2 Properties of Hemoglobin

Human hemoglobin is a tetramer produced by the reversible association of two pairs of globin chains. Normally, each molecule consists of two α chains and two non-α chains (β, γ, δ, ϵ). There are at least two known nonallelic normal structural variants of the γ chain, differing by one amino acid at position 136, called γ^{ala} and γ^{gly}. In the absence of α chains, tetramers of non-α chains may form (e.g., ϵ_4, a normal hemoglobin during early fetal life; β_4 or γ_4 in certain of the thalassemias). The globin chains are polypeptides of 141 (α) or 146 (non-α) amino acids in length, arranged in a series of straight stretches in the α-helical configuration, joined by short nonhelical regions. In the schematic model of a single globin monomer illustrated in Figure 8–1, the helical regions are designated by the letters A through H

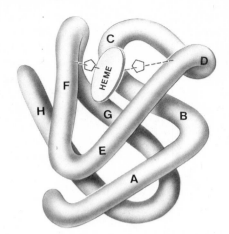

Fig. 8–1.—Model of a single globin molecule. The heme prosthetic group, with two critical interactions with hystidyl groups of the globin chain, are emphasized. $A-H$ = helical regions.

from the amino-terminal end of the polypeptide. The interior spaces of the hemoglobin tetramer contain only nonpolar amino acids, preserving a nonaqueous (hydrophobic) internal environment. Amino acids with polar side chains are exclusively directed at the external surface of the molecule.

Each globin chain possesses one tightly but reversibly bound prosthetic heme group. The heme group and its Fe^{++} atom are embedded, perpendicular to the surface, in a crevice formed by the E and F regions within the hydrophobic interior space of the mole-

Fig. 8–2.—The six coordinations (valences) of iron in hemoglobin.

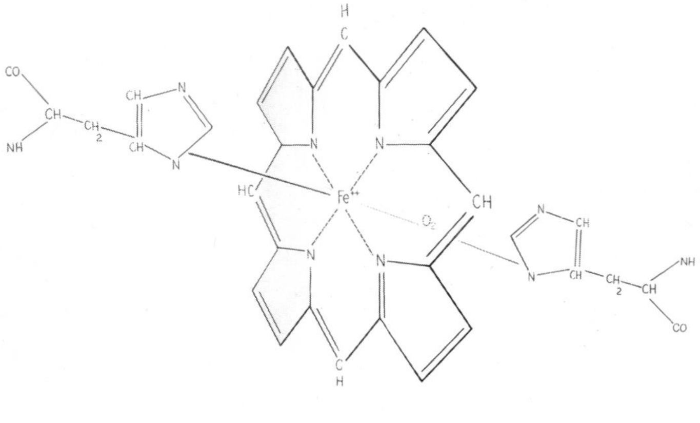

cule (see Fig. 8–1). This nonaqueous environment is essential to preserve the heme in its biologically active Fe^{++} form. The heme group forms a highly specific set of over 30 interactions with adjacent nonpolar amino acids. Two critical heme-globin interactions are mediated through valences of the Fe atom (Fig. 8–2). Iron has six coordinations (valences). Four of these interact with pyrrole nitrogen atoms and fix the iron in the porphyrin ring. The fifth valence involves the N of a histidyl residue in the F-helix, and the last bond, directed in the opposite direction, faces a histidine in the E-helix and contains the electron needed for the reversible transport of oxygen. These fifth and sixth coordinations of iron are of paramount importance to the preservation of heme in its reduced (Fe^{++} oxygen-transporting) rather than its oxidized (Fe^{+++} methemoglobin) form, which cannot transport oxygen, and to the stability of the structure of the hemoglobin molecule.

The four globin chains that form the hemoglobin tetramer are arranged so that two types of globin-globin interfaces are formed, the $\alpha_1\beta_1$ (or $\alpha_2\beta_2$) contact zone, and the $\alpha_1\beta_2$ (or $\alpha_2\beta_1$) contact (Fig. 8–3). The $\alpha_1\beta_1$ interface contributes principally to the structural

stability of the tetramer. There is little or no movement at this contact during oxygenation. The $\alpha_1\beta_2$ contact undergoes a large movement (about 13 degrees of rotation) during oxygenation-deoxygenation; this movement is essential for the normal oxygen affinity properties of hemoglobin.

8.2.1 OXYGEN TRANSPORT

The oxygen-dissociation curve of hemoglobin is sigmoid in configuration (Fig. 8–4). This relationship of oxygen content to oxygen tension (partial pressure of oxygen) permits efficient delivery of oxygen at the usual tissue oxygen tensions (around 40 mm Hg) and virtually complete saturation of hemoglobin at the normal oxygen tension of pulmonary alveolar capillaries (100 mm Hg). The sigmoid oxygen-dissociation curve is dependent upon so-called "heme-heme" interaction, the progressive enhancement of oxygen uptake as additional heme moieties become oxygenated. The most clear-cut fac-

Fig. 8–4.—Oxygen dissociation curve of hemoglobin. When the sigmoid curve is shifted to the left, oxygen is held more firmly by the hemoglobin; a shift to the right increases oxygen release. S_V = venous oxygen saturation; S_A = arterial oxygen saturation. Oxygen is released as blood goes from S_A (normal, 97%) to S_V (normal, 75%).

Fig. 8–3.—The hemoglobin tetramer: four globin chains and the two classes of globin-globin interfaces ($\alpha_1\beta_1$ type and $\alpha_1\beta_2$ type).

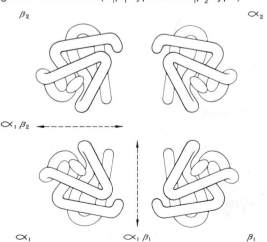

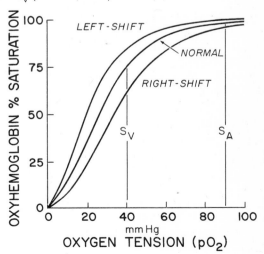

tor in this process is the physical movement of globin chains at the $\alpha_1\beta_2$ interface. Amino acid substitutions at this interface, which disturb this allosteric property of hemoglobin, produce abnormal oxygen-dissociation curves. Tetramers that contain only identical globin monomers (β_4 or γ_4) also have abnormal (high) oxygen affinity.

The oxygen affinity of hemoglobin (oxygen bound at a specified partial pressure) also is dependent on two additional factors:

1. *The Bohr effect,* which specifies that, as the pH is lowered, more oxygen will be released from hemoglobin (i.e., the oxygen-dissociation curve is shifted to the right). Tissue pH tends to be relatively low, and oxygen is efficiently released where it is metabolically required.

2. The intracellular concentration of certain organic phosphates, notably *2,3-diphosphoglycerate* (2,3-DPG). This molecule binds reversibly to the β chain of hemoglobin at the N-terminal end and profoundly modifies the position of the oxygen-dissociation curve. The curve is shifted progressively to the right (decreased O_2 affinity) as the molar ratio of 2,3-DPG:hemoglobin increases toward unity. The red cell concentration of 2,3-DPG, which is generated by the Rapaport-Luebering cycle of the Embden-Meyerhof pathway (see Fig. 7–1), is increased by hypoxia. An increase in 2,3-DPG of 1 mM/liter of red cells produces a shift in the p50 (the oxygen tension at which blood is 50% saturated) of the whole blood oxygen-dissociation curve of 3.8 mm Hg to the right. Thus, hypoxia itself creates the metabolic conditions for more oxygen delivery. The high oxygen affinity of HbF ($\alpha_2\gamma_2$) is due to the inability of this hemoglobin to bind 2,3-DPG.

8.3 Hemoglobin Variants

A gene for each of the normal globin chains (α, β, γ^{ala}, γ^{gly}, δ and ϵ) is inherited from each parent. Circumstantial evidence, derived from studies on the α-thalassemia syndromes (see section 8.7.6), raises the possibility that there may be more than one α globin structural gene in the normal human haploid genome. These structural genes, the hemoglobins to which they contribute and their time of appearance during fetal or postnatal life are illustrated in Table 1–1. Although the synthesis of each of these globin chains is under the control of separate genetic loci, the genes for β, γ and δ chains are closely linked. HbA is the major normal adult hemoglobin. HbA$_2$ is a minor adult hemoglobin normally accounting for less than 2.5–3% of hemoglobin. HbF is the major fetal hemoglobin and becomes a minor component (less than 1–2%) in adult blood. Hb Gower I and Gower II are normal but transient embryonic hemoglobins that disappear during gestation (see section 1.4).

Most pathologic genetic variants result from single amino acid substitutions in one of the normal globin chains. The hemoglobin tetramers formed by the variant globin plus the appropriate normal globin commonly are designated by a trivial name (a letter, often with an indication of the city of first discovery) and more strictly by an indication of the specific substitution. For example, sickle cell hemoglobin is abbreviated HbS; the globin composition is $\alpha_2\beta_2^s$ or, more precisely, $\alpha_2\beta_2^{6glu \rightarrow val}$, indicating that this pathologic hemoglobin consists of normal α chains plus β chains in which a valine has been substituted for the glutamine residue normally found at the sixth amino acid position from the N-terminal end. Each of the substituted globin variants thus represent an allelic form of one of the normal globin genetic loci. They may exist in either the heterozygous or homozygous state. At the β chain locus, for example, it is possible to recognize, clinically, individuals who are heterozygous for β^s and normal β (β^s/β^A); homozygous for the sickle cell gene (β^s/β^s); or doubly heterozygous for two β chain pathologic variants (e.g., β^s/β^c; β^c also may be designated $\beta^{6glu \rightarrow lys}$).

Many, but not all, amino acid substitutions result in net charge differences. For this reason hemoglobin electrophoresis has proved a powerful clinical and research tool for identification and diagnosis of variant hemoglobins. Some normal hemoglobins as well as pathologic variants are not readily identified or quantitated by these technics, at least under standard conditions. For example, HbF is not clearly distinguished from HbA by electrophoresis in the usual buffers. HbF is uniquely resistant to denaturation by alkali and this is routinely exploited as a method for determination of this normal hemoglobin component. Certain unstable hemoglobin variants that do not migrate uniquely on electrophoresis are detected by their precipitation when heated at 50 C.

8.3.1 Pathophysiology of the Hemoglobin Variants

Hemoglobin variants produce hematologic disease by three basic mechanisms, which are not mutually exclusive (Table 8 – 1):

1. Change in hemoglobin solubility due to substitutions at the surface of the molecule that produce abnormal interactions between adjacent hemoglobin tetramers.

2. Instability of the hemoglobin quaternary structure, resulting in spontaneous or drug-induced denaturation.

3. Abnormality of the oxygen-transport function.

On a world-wide basis, of the hemoglobin variants, only HbS and to a lesser degree HbC, both of which are pathogenic by the

TABLE 8 – 1. — EXAMPLES OF HEMOGLOBIN VARIANTS

CHARACTERISTICS	NAME	STRUCTURAL ALTERATION
Reduced solubility		
	S (sickle)	$\beta^{6 \ glu} \to val$
	C	$\beta^{6 \ glu} \to lys$
	C Harlem	$\beta^{6 \ glu} \to val$ and $\beta^{73 \ asp} \to asn$
Abnormal O$_2$ transport		
Increased O$_2$ affinity	Chesapeake	$\alpha^{92 \ arg} \to leu$
	Rainer	$\beta^{145 \ tyr} \to his$
	Hiroshima	$\beta^{143 \ his} \to asp$
	Tacoma	$\beta^{30 \ arg} \to ser$
	Zurich	$\beta^{63 \ his} \to arg$
	Gun Hill	deletion: $\beta^{93-97} \to O$
	Freiburg	deletion: $\beta^{23 \ val} \to O$
	H	β_4 (α-thalassemia)
	Barts	γ_4 (α-thalassemia)
Decreased O$_2$ affinity	Kansas	$\beta^{102 \ asn} \to thr$
	Hammersmith	$\beta^{42 \ phe} \to ser$
	Seattle	$\beta^{76 \ ala} \to glu$
	Torino	$\alpha^{43 \ phe} \to val$
Methemoglobins	M$_{Boston}$	$\alpha^{58 \ his} \to tyr$
	M$_{Iwate}$	$\alpha^{47 \ his} \to tyr$
	M$_{Saskatoon}$	$\beta^{63 \ his} \to tyr$
	M$_{Hyde \ Park}$	$\beta^{92 \ his} \to tyr$
Unstable molecules		
α Chain mutants	Torino	$\alpha^{43 \ phe} \to val$
β Chain mutants	Zurich	$\beta^{63 \ his} \to arg$
	Seattle	$\beta^{76 \ ala} \to glu$
	Genova	$\beta^{28 \ leu} \to pro$
	Hammersmith	$\beta^{42 \ phe} \to ser$
	Tacoma	$\beta^{30 \ arg} \to ser$
	Gun Hill	deletion: $\beta^{93-97} \to O$
	Freiburg	deletion: $\beta^{23 \ val} \to O$
	H	β_4

first mechanism, have a high incidence of significant morbidity. The other mutant globins have limited clinical importance statistically but have made major contributions to the elucidation of basic structure-function relationships in the hemoglobin molecule.

8.4 HbS Syndromes

The amino acid substitution, $\beta^{6glu \rightarrow val}$, results in a hemoglobin tetramer, $\alpha_2\beta_2^S$, which in the deoxygenated state is 50-fold less soluble than deoxyhemoglobin A. The β^S gene has an incidence of 5–20% in central and western African black populations and about 10% in the American black population. The balanced polymorphism exhibited by this gene has been speculatively attributed to resistance to Falciparum malaria conferred by the heterozygous β^S genotype. Diagnosis of homozygous HbS disease depends upon demonstrating sickling by in vitro deoxygenation and upon hemoglobin electrophoresis. HbS is the major hemoglobin, HbA is completely absent and there are variable amounts of HbF (generally about 5%).

Several hypothetical models that attempt to provide a molecular basis for the decreased solubility of deoxygenated HbS have been proposed. Whatever the final accepted mechanism, in homozygous HbS disease rigid, polymerized molecular aggregates form at reduced oxygen tensions within the physiologic range. These molecular "tactoids" profoundly alter red cell shape ("sickle" cell), fluidity and perhaps metabolic properties. Some red cells after repeated sickling transformations become irreversibly sickled and are subject to sequestration by the reticuloendothelial system. This process probably accounts for the life-long hemolytic anemia (ranging generally from 6–9 gm% hemoglobin) sustained by patients with homozygous HbS disease.

disease are subject to acute crises of ischemic tissue injury due to accelerated localized sickling that produces vascular stasis; progressive localized deoxygenation; more sickling and a vicious cycle that results in progressive vascular injury, pain and organ damage. These ischemic crises often are triggered by infections that alter local tissue perfusion and precipitate stasis, hypoxemia and red cell sickling. Ischemic crises may be reversible or may lead to infarction of the organ involved. Splenic infarction is a regular occurrence, and the splenomegaly found during childhood HbS disease invariably disappears due to repeated infarction of that organ. In the pediatric age, bone infarction involving the hands (dactylitis) is not uncommon and may mimic rheumatic fever symptoms. Necrosis of the heads of long bones, femora in particular, is more common in adults. Cerebrovascular complications are well documented, and pulmonary, renal and other organ involvement is a common adult manifestation.

The management of ischemic crises is supportive in nature, resting upon (1) a thorough search for and treatment of infection, (2) administration of fluids and (3) analgesia. Transfusions have been used to reduce the concentration of HbS and suppress endogenous HbS production, but the efficacy of this approach remains speculative. Anticoagulation has been advocated, but a role for coagulation mechanisms in HbS ischemic crisis is undocumented.

The use of cyanate, which forms covalent carbamyl linkages with globin chains, to reduce sickling and alleviate both the hemolytic anemia and ischemic crises, has been under investigation. The toxicity of this agent precludes clinical use. Other antisickling agents are presently under investigation.

8.4.1 ISCHEMIC CRISES

Intermittently, and for the moment unpredictably, patients with homozygous HbS

8.4.2 HYPOPLASTIC CRISES

Another less frequent but serious "crisis" in the natural history of sickle cell disease is the *hypoplastic crisis,* a transient episode of marrow failure, apparently triggered by certain intercurrent infections. In the face of vigorous hemolysis, such erythroid hypoplasia results rapidly in a potentially life-threatening decrease in the already low hemoglobin level. Reticulocytosis falls and the marrow shows diagnostic erythroid hypoplasia. Supportive management, with transfusion if needed, and a few days' time will almost always tide the patient over the transient danger.

The intense chronic erythropoietic activity in patients with homozygous S disease can deplete folic acid stores, and a megaloblastic component may be added to the hemolytic disease. Folic acid supplements are part of the usual treatment regimen for sickle cell anemia.

8.4.3 SICKLE CELL HETEROZYGOTES

The clinical expression of HbS is profoundly influenced by the presence of another hemoglobin in the affected red cell. Elevated HbF levels, for example, exert an ameliorating effect on HbS disease. The presence of HbA, which constitutes over 50% of the hemoglobin in the heterozygous sickle cell state (so-called sickle trait, β^A/β^S genetically), so depresses the sickling phenomenon that only under relatively extreme hypoxemic circumstances, perhaps coupled with severe acidosis or other predisposing metabolic states, are clinical manifestations observed. Almost invariably sickle cell trait is asymptomatic with respect to both anemia and ischemic crises.

Not all hemoglobins interact with HbS to suppress sickling, however. Most notable is HbC. HbC will co-polymerize extensively with deoxy-HbS. Although the disorder imposed by double heterozygosity for β^S and β^C (HbSC disease) may be somewhat milder in course than homozygous HbS disease, all of the serious complications are observed, including hemolytic anemia, ischemic crises, infarctions and a propensity for serious complications during pregnancy leading to increased fetal and maternal morbidity. Persistent splenomegaly is common in HbSC disease, unlike homozygous HbS. The combination of one gene for β^S and one for β-thalassemia produces a sickling disorder of variable severity, which is discussed in section 8.7.5.

8.5 Hemoglobin C Syndromes

The β^C globin allele ($\beta^{6glu \rightarrow lys}$) may be present in the homozygous form (β^C/β^C, called HbC disease) or heterozygous, with either the normal allele (β^C/β^A; HbC trait) or another pathologic β chain variant (e.g., β^C/β^S; see section 8.4.3). HbC trait, found in about 2% of the American black population, is invariably asymptomatic, although an increased number of target-shaped red cells may be detected in the peripheral blood smear. Homozygous HbC displays a mild hemolytic anemia with some potential for ischemic complications, especially of the femoral heads and optic vasculature. HbC is less soluble than HbA under conditions of increased ionic strength, but the precise pathogenesis of hemolysis remains obscure. There is no effect of deoxygenation on the physical properties of this hemoglobin.

8.6 Rare Hemoglobinopathies

Other amino acid substitutions, at internal loci if they are pathogenic, generally result in a change in oxygen transport and/or in physical instability of the hemoglobin tetramer.

8.6.1 METHEMOGLOBINS (HbM)

These variants (see Table 8–1) all result from substitutions that disturb the critical amino acid relationships surrounding the fifth and sixth coordinations of Fe^{++}. Of the five HbM variants known, four are substitutions of a tyrosine at one or the other of the two critical histidyl residues in the E- and F-helices of either the α or β globin chains (see

Figs. 8–1 and 8–2). In each case, the tyrosine side chain is long enough to accept permanently the electron that is normally used at the sixth coordination position of Fe^{++} for reversible oxygen binding. The methemoglobin (Fe^{+++} hemoglobin) so-formed cannot be reduced by the physiologic methemoglobin reductase system. The patient suffers from life-long cyanosis, present at birth if the mutant is an α chain allele, or appearing within 3–6 months of birth if it is a β mutant. The differential diagnosis of methemoglobinemia includes genetic deficiency of methemoglobin reductase (NADH-dependent diaphorase) and drug toxicity by agents that can oxidize heme, in addition to HbM variants.

8.6.2 Hemoglobins with Altered Oxygen Affinity

Amino acid substitutions that disturb the $\alpha_1\beta_2$ interface (see Fig. 8–3) may affect those allosteric movements that are necessary for normal oxygen affinity. Of the known variants of this type (see Table 8–1), most are high-affinity hemoglobins; they produce tissue hypoxia due to inefficient oxygen release and polycythemia (elevated red cell mass) due to increased erythropoietin production. Some have low oxygen affinity, displaying cyanosis and anemia, but patients generally are asymptomatic since tissue oxygenation is adequate. Many of the hemoglobins of this class also are highly unstable molecules and may produce hemolytic anemia on that basis. The differential diagnosis of polycythemia includes, in addition to these rare hemoglobins, polycythemia vera (one of the myeloproliferative diseases; Chapter 11), chronic hypoxia of cardiorespiratory origin and increased erythropoietin production due to local renal hypoxia or autonomous production in neoplastic tissues. These will be discussed in Chapter 11.

8.6.3 Unstable Hemoglobins

These variants (see Table 8–1) comprise a large group of amino acid substitutions in α and β globin chains, each of which results in an unstable tetramer that denatures spontaneously or when exposed to oxidant drugs of the sort implicated in G-6-PD deficiency. Substitutions that (1) destabilize the heme moiety in its hydrophobic pocket, (2) introduce polar amino acids into the interior of the hemoglobin molecule, (3) alter the helical configuration of critical regions or (4) alter the $\alpha_1\beta_1$ interface are responsible for these unstable hemoglobins, many of which display abnormal oxygen affinity as well.

Chronic hemolytic anemia of variable severity, often accelerated by drugs or infection and displaying Heinz body formation, is typical of these disorders. The abnormal hemoglobin may or may not be distinguished by electrophoresis, but its presence is demonstrated by heat precipitation at 50 C for 60 minutes. Management consists principally of avoiding oxidant drugs; splenectomy has been of indifferent value.

8.7 The Thalassemias

The thalassemias constitute a group of hereditary disorders of hemoglobin synthesis that share certain common clinical manifestations including hypochromic anemia with marked poikilocytosis, Heinz body-type intraerythrocytic precipitates, ineffective erythropoiesis and accelerated hemolysis. In each of the thalassemias, the principal biochemical manifestation is a partial or complete, but always selective, deficiency in the synthesis of one of the major globin chains. In the normal erythroblast and reticulocyte, α and β globin chains are produced in roughly equal amounts. Thalassemic red cells are characterized by an excess of the unaffected globin chain, which is produced at a normal rate. β-Thalassemia refers to those disorders characterized by deficient β chain synthesis; α-thalassemia results from deficient α chain production. Each of these categories includes variants that differ in severity and very probably in the precise molecular mechanism leading to defective globin synthesis. The thalassemias differ from the hemoglobinopathies proper in that there is as yet no evidence for a simple amino acid substitution in any globin chain affected by a thalassemia gene. However, more complex structural abnormalities of the globin genes, including unequal crossing-over between β and δ genes (Hb Lepore) and a chain termination defect (Hb Constant Spring), are definitely associated with thalassemia-like syndromes. In the few patients with α- or β-thalassemia who have been studied in great detail, the present evidence indicates a quantitative deficiency in the amount of specific (e.g., α or β) globin mRNA in the affected erythroid cells. Whether or not all thalassemias display this same type of molecular deficiency, as well as the nature of the genetic defects that result in selective globin mRNA deficiency, has yet to be determined.

The clinical effects of insufficient synthesis of specific globin chains depend upon the severity of the defect in hemoglobin production, upon the degree of imbalance of α and β globin chains in the red cells, upon the specific chain that is deficient and upon more indirect but not less serious consequences of the genetic disorder, including the deleterious effects of chronic life-long anemia and disordered iron metabolism.

8.7.1 β-Thalassemia Syndromes

The gene or genes for β-thalassemia are found in the highest incidence among Mediterranean, Middle Eastern, Indian and Far Eastern populations. Once again, a relationship to the distribution of Falciparum malaria has been suggested but remains unproved.

Genetic evidence indicates that the β-thalassemia gene is closely linked with the β globin chain structural gene. Furthermore, at least two variants of the β-thalassemia syndrome can be recognized: (1) β-thalassemia in which the thalassemia gene is associated with total lack of synthesis of any β globin (so-called β^0), and (2) β-thalassemia with partial suppression of β globin synthesis (β^+). Evidence for these two variants comes from the study of patients who are doubly heterozygous for β-thalassemia and for a β chain structural mutant such as HbS (genotype β^{thal}/β^S). Electrophoresis of the hemoglobin from some patients of this genetic constitution reveals no HbA whatsoever—only HbS and the minor hemoglobins, F and A_2. The thalassemia gene in these patients is of the β^0 variety. Other double heterozygotes display a small but definite amount of HbA (5–30%), in addition to a major HbS component (60% or greater), HbA_2 and HbF. These patients have the β^+ variant of the β-thalassemia gene. They may be distinguished from simple HbS heterozygotes (S-trait), because in S-trait the quantity of HbS is always *less than* 50% of the total. Erythroid cells from patients homozygous for β^0-thalassemia contain no detectable HbA and synthesize no detectable β globin, whereas cells from β^+-thalassemic homozygotes may contain small amounts of HbA, and a low level of β chain synthesis can be detected. Family studies are, of course, invaluable in establishing the genetic basis of the clinical features of patients with the thalassemia variants.

Historically the β-thalassemias have been classified according to clinical severity and the terms, thalassemia major, intermedia, minor and minima, will be found in the literature. Now that the genetic basis of these disorders is reasonably well understood, it is far preferable to refer to heterozygous and homozygous β-thalassemia wherever possible.

8.7.2 Pathophysiology of β-Thalassemia

The pathophysiology of the anemia and ineffective erythropoiesis in homozygous β-thalassemia (Cooley's anemia; Mediterranean anemia) is complex; two principal contributory factors are as follows:

1. Decreased synthesis of HbA due to deficient β globin mRNA and insufficient β globin production, resulting in poorly hemoglobinized red cells that have a shortened survival in the peripheral blood.

2. A relative excess of α chains, which cannot form stable $\alpha_2\beta_2$ tetramers. Instead,

the excess α chains form insoluble precipitates of denatured α globin. These precipitates result in accelerated intramedullary destruction of erythroblasts, i.e., ineffective erythropoiesis. Some of the excess α chains may combine with γ chains to form HbF and with δ chains to form HbA_2; indeed the rate of γ chain synthesis is moderately elevated in the commonest variants of β-thalassemia. However, neither γ nor δ chains are synthesized in sufficient numbers to replace the deficient β chains and prevent denaturation and precipitation of excess α chains in the form of Heinz bodies.

8.7.3 CLINICAL FEATURES OF HOMOZYGOUS β-THALASSEMIA

The disease can be detected early in infancy, as the γ chain synthesis characteristic of fetal life subsides and β chain production fails to take over normally. Red cell morphologic stigmata often can be recognized by 6 weeks of age; these include severe hypochromia, anisocytosis, target cells, poikilocytosis, basophilic stippling and, in time, nucleated red cells (NRBC) in the peripheral blood. Red cell inclusion bodies are revealed by supravital staining and resemble Heinz bodies. The number of NRBC and Heinz bodies usually increases after splenectomy.

Poor growth and development due to chronic anemia—as well as skeletal changes involving skull, long bones and hands due to intense but ineffective marrow erythroid hyperplasia—are characteristic. Affected children are subject to recurrent infections but the most vexing of all complications is the inevitable development of severe hemosiderosis. This is due in part to iron deposition from transfused blood, but anemia itself appears to accelerate iron uptake and its deposition in parenchymal tissue. The most devastating site of siderosis is the myocardium, which leads to both conduction defects and heart failure. Heart disease is a major factor in the death of affected individuals in

childhood or early adult life. Some patients survive longer, but as yet no genetic or physiologic basis for prolonged survival has been ascertained.

The clinical consequences of intense ineffective erythropoiesis from an early age are striking: (1) erythroid hyperplasia, causing severe medullary expansion and the skeletal lesions described; (2) extensive extramedullary erythropoiesis, producing massive hepatosplenomegaly and even lymphadenopathy and (3) accelerated bilirubin production, predisposing to biliary tract disease.

The hemoglobin electrophoresis pattern in homozygous β-thalassemia is characterized by variable amounts of HbF and HbA_2 and by the presence or absence of HbA, depending on whether the thalassemia genes are $β^+$ or $β^0$. HbF can range from 10–90% of the total hemoglobin. The γ chains produced are structurally normal. HbF is distributed in a heterogeneous manner among the red cells in β-thalassemia, as determined by a cytologic technic. Some cells may contain relatively large amounts of HbF, others only small amounts. There is some evidence that the high F cells have longer in vivo survival, but the over-all severity of the disease does not correlate well with HbF levels. δ Chain production in homozygous β-thalassemia is variable, and HbA_2 constitutes from 1–4% of the hemoglobin.

The management of children with β-thalassemia is difficult and fraught with clinical dilemmas. Growth and mental retardation may be ameliorated by regular blood transfusions, but this accelerates the development of life-threatening hemosiderosis. The use of iron-chelating agents for the prevention of siderosis is under intensive investigation, but success to date has not been impressive. Splenectomy is considered when rapid splenic sequestration of transfused red cells seriously increases the rate of transfusion requirement. The risk of serious postsplenectomy sepsis in young children usually dictates postponement of this procedure until as late in childhood as possible.

8.7.4 HETEROZYGOUS β-THALASSEMIA

Thalassemia trait or minima is generally asymptomatic, without anemia, but displays a variable degree of thalassemic red cell morphology in the peripheral blood smear. A mistaken diagnosis of iron deficiency might be entertained but would be eliminated by finding normal plasma iron values and adequate-to-elevated marrow iron stores. Some heterozygotes (so-called thalassemia minor) display a mild anemia, with evidence of fairly well-compensated hemolysis and ineffective erythropoiesis. The principal diagnostic feature of this genetic disorder is an elevated level of HbA_2 (about 5% compared to a mean normal HbA_2 of about 2.5%). HbF levels are normal. There is unbalanced synthesis of α and β chains in the heterozygote due to decreased β globin production, but the defect, due to single gene dose, is not sufficient to initiate the severe pathogenic mechanisms seen in homozygous β-thalassemia.

8.7.5 SYNDROMES RELATED TO β-THALASSEMIA

As already noted, when a gene for β-thalassemia is inherited from one parent and a $β^s$ gene from the other (HbS/β-thalassemia double heterozygosity), the biochemical lesion produced is the sum of both genetic defects. HbA production is directed solely by the $β^{thal}$ gene. If it is $β^0$, no HbA can be produced; if it is $β^+$, some HbA is synthesized but always less than 50% of the total. The remainder is HbS plus the small elevation of HbA_2 characteristic of thalassemia trait. Clinically the disease resembles the HbS disorders, and the severity, modulated by the amount of HbA produced, varies from asymptomatic (as HbS trait) to severe with ischemic crises and hemolytic anemia, as in sickle cell disease.

A thalassemia gene that directs deficient synthesis of both β and δ globin chains (δβ-thalassemia) has been identified in both heterozygous and homozygous form in Mediterranean, black and Far Eastern populations. The clinical pattern is typically thalassemic; in the homozygous state the hemoglobin pattern is entirely HbF.

It has already been noted that the globin chains made under the control of the β-thalassemia genes are normal in amino acid sequence. Exceptions to this rule are known, both for β- and for α-thalassemia-like disorders. *Hb Lepore* is one such: there is strong evidence that Hb Lepore represents the product of an unequal cross-over between the closely linked structural δ and β loci (Fig. 8–5). Hb Lepore thus represents the N-terminal portion of a δ chain fused genetically to the C-terminal end of a β chain. This genetic fusion product behaves in a simple mendelian fashion, like all structural genes. In the heterozygous state patients are asymptomatic but show the morphologic red cell stigmata of thalassemia trait. Hemoglobins A, F, Lepore and A_2 are produced. Clinically the homozygous state resembles homozygous β-thalassemia in virtually all respects; the hemoglobin pattern reveals HbF (about 75%) and Hb Lepore, with no detectable HbA or

Fig. 8–5.—Gene for Hb Lepore, the product of an unequal cross-over event involving the adjacent β and δ chain loci.

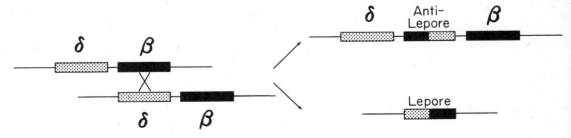

HbA_2. Recently patients with hemoglobins that have the properties of an "anti-Lepore" hemoglobin (i.e., the alternative fusion product of the unequal cross-over; see Fig. 8–5) have been identified. These patients possess normal β and δ genes in addition to the fusion gene, and there are no clinical manifestations of thalassemia.

There is a group of widespread hereditary conditions called *hereditary persistence of fetal hemoglobin* (HPFH) in which β and δ chain synthesis is completely (black type) or partially (Greek type) suppressed by the mutation but, unlike the $\delta\beta$-thalassemias, γ chains are synthesized at a high level, sufficient to compensate completely for the deficient β and δ chains. There are no significant clinical findings other than a mild polycythemia in the homozygotes (due to the increased oxygen affinity of HbF). HbF is distributed in a homogeneous fashion in the affected red cells (unlike the pattern in the true β-thalassemias). The uniform distribution of elevated HbF in HPFH probably accounts for the mild clinical manifestations observed in the double heterozygote, HPFH/β^s, compared with β^{thal}/β^s.

8.7.6 α-THALASSEMIA SYNDROMES

Analogous to the β-thalassemias, these disorders are the consequence of partial or complete suppression of normal α chain synthesis. Since α chains are components of HbA, HbA_2 and HbF, detection of α-thalassemia heterozygotes is not based simply on hemoglobin electrophoresis patterns, as in β-thalassemia heterozygotes. Furthermore, the genetic interpretation of the α-thalassemias is complicated by two factors:

1. There is a strong possibility that the α chain structural locus is reduplicated (at least in many populations) and possibly even translocated (i.e., no longer closely linked.)

2. There is some evidence that there may be two α-thalassemia genes; α-thalassemia$_1$, which directs total suppression of α chain synthesis, and α-thalassemia$_2$, which determines a less severe deficiency of α chain synthesis. The major α-thalassemia syndromes, it is currently speculated, are the consequence either of permutations of these two allelic α-thalassemic genes or, alternatively, of deletion or inactivation of one or both of the putative α chain structural loci. Three principal α-thalassemia syndromes can be identified.

The first of these, *hydrops fetalis with Hb Bart's*, is the most severe form of α-thalassemia. No α chains are produced, and the disease is most simply considered to be the result either of homozygosity for the α-thalassemia$_1$ gene or deletion of all α structural genes. α Chains are required for normal hemoglobin production even in fetal life, and affected conceptuses consequently are severely anemic in utero and are born dead. The major hemoglobins found in cord blood are Hb Bart's (γ_4), which constitutes 80–90% of hemoglobin, and HbH (β_4). The parents of such conceptuses are α-thalassemia heterozygotes.

HbH disease, the second principal syndrome, is recognized by a thalassemia-like hematologic picture, with intraerythrocytic inclusions due to precipitation of unstable HbH (β_4). The hemoglobin pattern reveals HbA, 10–30% HbH and small amounts of Hb Bart's. There always is anemia, and hepatosplenomegaly and skeletal changes are frequent. The disease may be as severe as full-blown β-thalassemia at one extreme and compatible with normal life at the other end of the broad clinical spectrum. It is hypothesized that HbH disease is the consequence of either double heterozygosity for the α-thalassemia$_1$ and α-thalassemia$_2$ genes, or deletion of several but not all α structural genes.

Detection of simple heterozygotes for α-thalassemia, α-*thalassemia trait*, the third of the syndromes, is difficult except in the parents of documented Hb Bart's hydrops fetalis abortuses. These parents display no anemia but mild thalassemic red cell morphology. When appropriate laboratory facilities are available, a study of the rates of synthesis of α and β globin chains by reticulocytes from suspected carriers can be used to confirm the presence of α-thalassemia trait.

A full understanding of the α-thalassemia syndromes awaits more complete elucidation of the genetic mechanisms.

9

White Blood Cells: Structure, Kinetics and Function

9.1 Introduction

THE HUMAN WHITE BLOOD CELL SYSTEM is composed of several cell types: granulocytes, lymphocytes, plasma cells and monocytes. The major function of granulocytes is host defense; these cells are active in phagocytosis of foreign particles including bacteria. Disorders of granulocytopoiesis that interfere with either the number or function of granulocytes lead to increased risk of bacterial infection and decreased host response to foreign matter. Lymphocytes and plasma cells perform significant functions in immunologic reactions, including humoral antibody formation and cellular immunity. Defects in the production or function of these cells result in abnormal host responses. Monocytes also are active in the body's phagocytic and immunologic response to foreign materials or infections. Intact WBC function is therefore necessary for normal humoral and cellular responses to infectious agents and foreign materials.

9.2 Granulocytes

9.2.1 MORPHOLOGIC CHARACTERISTICS

Granulocytes are recognized in circulating blood and bone marrow by their characteristic morphologic appearance (Figs. 9–1 and 9–2). The more immature cells in the granulocytic (myeloid, myelocytic) series normally are found only in the bone marrow.

9.2.1.1 MYELOBLAST.—The earliest recognizable myeloid cell, the myeloblast, contains a large nucleus with scant blue cytoplasm. The nuclear chromatin is in fine

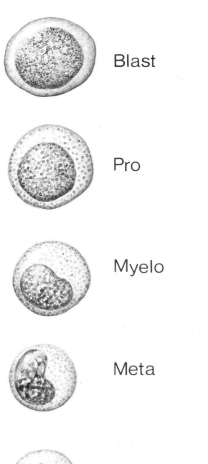

Blast

Pro

Myelo

Meta

Band

Poly

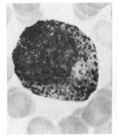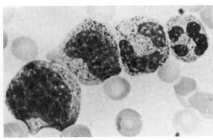

Fig. 9–1.—Left, normal bone marrow granulocytic elements (neutrophilic). Blast = myeloblast; Pro = promyelocyte; Myelo = myelocyte; Meta = metamyelocyte; Band = band form; Poly = polymorphonuclear neutrophil. **Above,** granulocyte maturation. From left to right, a promyelocyte, myelocyte, metamyelocyte and partially segmented and fully segmented neutrophilic polymorphonuclear granulocytes.

Fig. 9–2.—Normal leukocytes. **A,** neutrophilic granulocyte *(upper right);* monocyte *(lower left).* **B,** small lymphocyte.

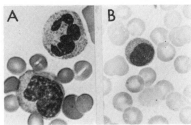

strands. With Wright's stain, the nucleus appears reddish purple and contains one or more nucleoli, which stain light blue or gray.

9.2.1.2. PROMYELOCYTE.—The next recognizable cell stage in granulocyte maturation is the promyelocyte. The nuclear chromatin is somewhat more clumped than that of the myeloblast. Nucleoli persist and the cytoplasm contains large azurophilic (red to purple) granules that overlie both nucleus and cytoplasm. These so-called primary granules contain a variety of lysosomal enzymes including acid hydrolases and myeloperoxidase. The presence of myeloperoxidase in immature myeloid precursors permits their recognition with use of specific stains for this enzyme.

9.2.1.3 MYELOCYTE.—The progeny of promyelocytes are myelocytes, characterized by further increase in the clumping of nuclear chromatin, loss of nucleoli and the appearance of definitive granules in the cytoplasm. Each of the granulocytic elements is characterized by unique definitive granules at the myelocyte stage. In the neutrophilic granulocytes, these granules are fine and pink on Wright's stain; their appearance varies somewhat from smear to smear. The granules are rich in the enzymes, alkaline phosphatase and lysozyme; they do not contain large amounts of acid hydrolases or myeloperoxidase. In eosinophilic granulocytes, the granules are larger, refractile and deeper pink or red. These granules contain basic proteins and peroxidase. Basophilic granulocytes have large, deep blue granules, which contain great amounts of histamine and heparin. The myelocyte is the last proliferating cell stage in granulopoiesis.

9.2.1.4 METAMYELOCYTE.—These cells are distinguished from myelocytes by their smaller size, more pronounced condensation of chromatin and a prominent indentation of the nucleus. The number of definitive granules increases during this phase. The metamyelocyte matures without cell division to become a band form.

9.2.1.5 BAND FORMS.—The band form is smaller than the metamyelocyte, and the nucleus now has a characteristic elongated but not yet lobulated form.

9.2.1.6 POLYMORPHONUCLEAR GRANULOCYTES.—The final stage in granulocytic development is the production of mature granulocytes containing a segmented nucleus. The nuclear segments are connected by fine filaments, and the cytoplasm contains definitive granules. Eosinophilic, basophilic and neutrophilic granulocytes are distinguished by their characteristic granules: in mature neutrophils the granules are fine and usually reddish pink; in eosinophils the granules are larger, refractile and pink to red; in basophils the granules are large and stain deep blue. Mature neutrophilic granulocytes, also termed polymorphonuclear neutrophils (PMN), usually contain two to four lobes. Hypersegmented PMN containing five or more lobes are characteristically found in megaloblastic anemias. In the PMN of females an ovoid mass of blue-staining material resembling a drumstick may be seen projecting from a nuclear segment. This is the Barr body, representing X chromosome material. Normally, only segmented granulocytes and a few band forms circulate in the peripheral blood. The presence of granulocytes that are more immature than band forms calls attention to accelerated or disordered granulopoiesis.

The *Pelger-Huët anomaly* is an inherited or acquired defect in granulocytes in which there is partial or complete failure of segmentation of granulocyte nuclei.

The polymorphonuclear granulocytic cells in peripheral blood and bone marrow must be distinguished from the lymphocytic and monocytic elements (see Figs. 9–1 and 9–2). The lymphocytes (see section 9.3) are most easily identified by their clear light blue cytoplasm, which contains a few azurophilic granules. Lymphocyte chromatin is characteristically clumped and the nucleus is either round or somewhat indented. Monocytes are larger than PMN, the nuclear chromatin is not as clumped as in lymphocytes and the nucleus is usually folded, although not segmented as in PMN. The monocyte cytoplasm is usually bluish gray, with small red granules uniformly distributed, having a so-called ground glass appearance. Plasma cells have a deep blue-staining cytoplasm with a clear area often present adjacent to the nucleus (perinuclear halo). The nucleus is usually round or somewhat indented and contains clumped chromatin, occasionally in a configuration resembling the spokes of a wheel. Plasma cells are rarely found in the circulation under normal circumstances.

9.2.2 EVALUATION OF WBC MORPHOLOGY

Since the staining characteristics of WBC may vary from slide to slide, the following scheme may be helpful in evaluating white cell morphology.

1. Find an area of the smear in which the red cells are not overlapping and the white cells are well stained and clearly seen.

2. Identify a typical PMN and note its cytoplasmic staining characteristics, especially the color and texture of the granules.

3. Identify a typical lymphocyte and note its cytoplasmic staining characteristics.

4. Identify other neutrophils by the similarity of the cytoplasm to that of typical PMN. Define the more immature granulocytes by differences in nuclear characteristics.

5. Identify monocytes by the differences in cytoplasmic staining between these cells and typical lymphocytes and PMN and by the presence of folded nuclei. The normal percentages of neutrophils, lymphocytes and monocytes, as well as eosinophils and basophils, are provided in the Appendix.

9.2.3 GRANULOCYTE METABOLISM

DNA synthesis and mitosis occur only in myeloblasts, promyelocytes and early myelocytes; RNA and protein synthesis are present at all stages of maturation but are most active in more immature cells. Granulocytes depend largely on glycolysis for their energy supply, using glucose and generating large amounts of lactic acid. Although enzymes of the tricarboxylic acid cycle are present in these cells, they contain few mitochondria and relatively little oxidative phosphorylation activity. Lipid biosynthesis is quite active at early stages of maturation and can be demonstrated by the incorporation of radioactively labeled acetate into lipid. Transcobalamin I, a vitamin B_{12}-binding protein, is present in and released from granulocytes. The serum level of transcobalamin I correlates with the mass of granulocytes in the body. Two enzymes of major importance are found in relatively large quantities in granulocytes:

1. *Myeloperoxidase,* abundant in the primary granules of granulocytes, which also contain other lysosomal enzymes capable of digesting foreign particles and bacteria. Myeloperoxidase can be identified by specific staining technics. When immature cells cannot be accurately identified as lymphocytes or myelocytes, the stain for peroxidase may be useful in defining the granulocytic origin of the cells.

2. *Alkaline phosphatase,* present in the definitive granules of granulocytic cells and which can be quantitated by specific histochemical stains. The amount of alkaline phosphatase present in mature granulocytes is useful in the differential diagnosis of certain abnormalities in the myeloid series, the myeloproliferative syndromes.

9.2.4 GRANULOCYTE FUNCTION

The metabolic activity of granulocytes is markedly increased as they participate in their major function, the phagocytosis of particles or bacteria. Increases in anaerobic and aerobic glycolysis, glycogenolysis, lipid synthesis and hydrogen peroxide production occur. The process of phagocytosis by PMN involves several steps:

1. Opsonins, including Ig, components of the complement system and other factors in serum, interact with foreign substances; the opsonization process and the presence of divalent cations enhance phagocytosis. The precise role of neutrophil mobility (chemotaxis) is unclear. In any event,

2. Opsonized particles become adherent to PMN in the area of injury or at the location of foreign substances.

3. Activation of contractile proteins and microtubules in the cytoplasm of phagocytic cells may be involved in pseudopod formation and invagination of the plasma membrane, resulting in ingestion of adherent particles and enclosure within membrane-lined vacuoles (phagocytic vacuoles).

4. Lysosomes, containing hydrolytic enzymes, fuse with the phagocytic vacuole.

5. Hydrolytic enzymes, released into the phagocytic vacuole, digest the foreign materials. No hydrolytic enzymes escape into the granulocyte cytoplasm outside of the vacuole. The precise mechanism of bacterial killing in granulocytes is a subject of considerable debate; the generation of hydrogen peroxide and other oxides as well as iodination of bacteria in the vacuoles may contribute to this process. Generation of hydrogen peroxide can be recognized cytochemically with nitrotetrazolium blue dye (NTB). Normal PMN develop a blue color in the presence of NTB when adequate hydrogen peroxide generation occurs.

9.2.5 CONGENITAL DEFECTS OF GRANULOCYTE STRUCTURE AND FUNCTION

Over the past several years, many congenital and acquired defects of neutrophils that result in abnormal phagocytosis and deficient bacterial killing have been described. These abnormalities reflect the complexity of the process of phagocytosis and provide insight into the many steps necessary for normal neutrophil function. Defects in neutrophil mobility, granule formation and enzymatic activity have all been shown to be responsible for abnormal phagocytosis and increased infections.

Chronic granulomatous disease is an inherited disorder, probably X-linked, seen in children and characterized by recurrent infections due to both gram-positive and gram-negative organisms with low grade pathogenicity. Eczema, hepatosplenomegaly, lymphadenopathy and granuloma formation occur. The cellular defect results in defective bactericidal action and is associated with decreased generation of hydrogen peroxide. Phagocytosis, phagocytic granule formation and lysosomal function appear normal. Reduction of NTB is deficient in the neutrophils of patients with chronic granulomatous disease (a negative NTB test).

Myeloperoxidase deficiency has been described in some patients with fungal infections, especially candidiasis. However, normal individuals also have been identified with this defect. Thus, the relationship between myeloperoxidase deficiency and increased susceptibility to infection is not yet clearly established.

Chediak-Higashi syndrome is an autosomal recessive inherited disorder associated with abnormal granulation of granulocytes, partial albinism and photophobia due to decreased or absent uveal pigment. Large blue peroxidase-positive cytoplasmic inclusions, resulting from abnormal development of primary granules, are found in granulocyte precursors and mature PMN. The defective primary granules are responsible for inadequate bacterial killing and are accompanied by defective phagocytosis. Consequently there is an increased incidence of infection. The disorder also is associated with histiocytic infiltration of the spleen, liver, lymph nodes and other organs, and pancytopenia occurs late in the disease. The disorder appears to be a generalized defect in granule formation affecting many tissues beside the hematopoietic cells. Neurologic complications are common. The disease is usually fatal at an early age.

The *May-Hegglin anomaly* is an inherited disorder associated with thrombocytopenia, giant platelets and blue-staining cytoplasmic inclusions in granulocytes, resembling so-called Döhle bodies. A variable bleeding tendency may be the major clinical manifestation. Döhle bodies, which principally contain RNA, also are found in PMN in association with infection, certain drugs and normal pregnancy.

In the *Alder-Reilly anomaly*, a recessively inherited disorder, small purplish granules or "bodies" are present in neutrophils. These granules, larger than the "toxic" granules accompanying infections, also are seen in patients with the Hurler syndrome, the Hunter syndrome and some other forms of dwarfism. Similar inclusions also are present in lymphocytes and monocytes. The Alder-Reilly bodies do not appear to interfere with granulocyte function.

In the *lazy-leukocyte syndrome* (as described in several children) there is an increase in infections associated with severe neutropenia. The bone marrow contains normal numbers of mature neutrophils that display normal neutrophil morphology, mobility and phagocytic capacity. However, these neutrophils show defective chemotactic responses to opsonized particles, which may account for the clinical manifestations.

9.2.6 GRANULOCYTE KINETICS

Granulocyte production normally takes place in the bone marrow. The multipotential hematopoietic stem cell under appropriate conditions differentiates to give rise to the earliest morphologically recognizable granulocytic precursor, the myeloblast.

Proliferating or dividing cells go through a characteristic cell cycle including both DNA synthesis (S phase) and mitosis (M) (Fig. 9–3). Two other stages of the cell cycle have been defined: G_1 is the stage of the cell cycle preceding DNA synthesis; G_2 is the stage following DNA synthesis and G_0 is the stage defined for resting cells that are not in cell cycle. When cells are in cycle, they pass through G_1, S, G_2 and M consecutively. In measurements of parameters of the cell cycle, tritiated thymidine is used as a label for the synthesis of DNA. The number of proliferating cells, (i.e., the number of cells in cell cycle during any period of time) can be measured by counting the number of cells that have incorporated labeled thymidine into their DNA by radioautography. The only granulocyte elements capable of DNA synthesis and mitosis are myeloblasts, promyelocytes and myelocytes. These cells comprise the proliferating pool of granulocytic cells and are normally restricted to the bone marrow (Fig. 9–4). Myeloblasts represent less than 5% of the total bone marrow granulocytes, promyelocytes 5–10% and myelocytes 10–15%. Thus, the cells capable of proliferation represent 20–30% of the total marrow granulocyte pool. The rest of the granulocytic cells in the bone marrow are maturing but nonproliferating metamyelocytes, bands and PMN. They form the major

Fig. 9–3.—Cell cycle kinetics. **A,** diagram of cell cycle. G_0 = resting phase; G_1 = phase preceding DNA synthesis; S = phase of DNA synthesis; G_2 = phase following DNA synthesis; M = mitosis. **B,** changes in DNA content/cell at different phases of cell cycle. 2C = diploid chromosome number (normal DNA content); 4c = twice 2C.

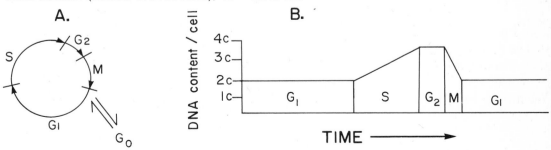

GRANULOCYTE   MATURATION

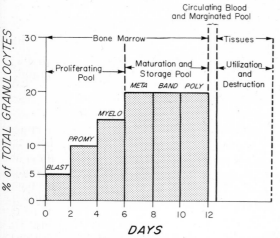

Fig. 9–4.—Granulocyte kinetics and pools. The abscissa in days indicates that a blast cell undergoes maturation to a polymorphonuclear leukocyte in an average of 12 days. Less than 1 day is spent by granulocytes released from the bone marrow in peripheral blood before utilization and destruction in the tissues. Blasts, promyelocytes and myelocytes are the only proliferating cells. After this stage there is further maturation as well as storage of granulocytes. The ordinate indicates the approximate percentage of the total granulocytes in the bone marrow at different stages of maturation.

storage pool of granulocytes in the body. The normal time required for development from the myeloblast stage until release into the circulation is 8–14 days, as determined by isotope-labeling studies. Under normal conditions only PMN and a few bands egress from the bone marrow. This is presumably due to the relative rigidity of immature granulocytes, which prevent their passage into the circulation. The peripheral blood contains a relatively small pool of mature neutrophils compared to the marrow pool (see Fig. 9–4).

The proliferative capacity of granulocytic cells can be determined by several methods:

1. The *mitotic index*. This is a measurement of the percentage of granulocytic cells in metaphase. It gives a rough estimate of

proliferation. Usually less than 1% of myeloid precursors in bone marrow is in mitotic metaphase at any instant.

2. The *labeling index*. When ^{3}H-thymidine is incubated with normal bone marrow cells, 10–50% of myeloblasts is labeled (i.e., is in cell cycle). The percentage of cells of a given type in cell cycle is the labeling index and is another measure of the proliferative capacity. Myeloblasts, promyelocytes and myelocytes are labeled, whereas the more differentiated granulocytic elements are not.

3. *Generation time*. This is defined as the interval required for proliferating cells to complete a single cycle. One method for evaluating the generation time of granulocytes is to expose bone marrow, in vitro or in vivo, to tritiated thymidine for a short time (pulse label) and by radioautography to follow the subsequent appearance of ^{3}H-thymidine-labeled mitoses. The first mitoses following the pulse of ^{3}H-thymidine will not be labeled, since these cells were in G_2 during the labeling period. Subsequently, labeled mitoses will appear as cells that were in S during the pulse enter mitosis. The number of labeled mitoses will increase to a maximum and then begin to decline as the cells that were in G_1 during the labeling begin to enter mitosis. The labeled cells will enter a second cycle and the proportion of labeled mitoses will once again increase and reach a second maximum. The generation time can be calculated from the interval between the two waves of labeled mitoses. Although there are significant technical difficulties in interpretation of measurements of the generation time of granulocytes, the generation time is approximately 24 hours for normal myelocyte precursors. The range is between 15 and 64 hours.

9.2.7 MARGINATED GRANULOCYTE POOL

When mature granulocytes enter the circulating blood, approximately 50% are immediately sequestered along vessel walls; these constitute the marginated granulocyte pool.

The presence of such a marginated pool can be demonstrated by labeling autologous granulocytes with radioactive diisofluorophosphate (DF^{32}P) and reinjecting them into the circulation. Approximately half of the labeled granulocytes fail to appear in the circulation. This is not due to damage to the ^{32}P-labeled cells, since these granulocytes can be recovered by subsequent injection of epinephrine or by exercise. DF^{32}P also can be used to measure the total blood granulocyte pool (TBGP) by determining the dilution of DF^{32}P label after reinjection of cells into the circulation.

9.2.8 CIRCULATING GRANULOCYTE LIFE SPAN

The loss of DF^{32}P-labeled granulocytes from the circulation can be used to determine the t$^{1/2}$ of granulocytes in the circulation, taking into account the marginated granulocyte pool. Using this measurement, it has been demonstrated that granulocytes have an extremely short life span in peripheral blood, with an average t$^{1/2}$ of 6.7 hours before they enter the tissues where they are either utilized, stored or destroyed. The pulmonary circulation represents a major site of sequestration of granulocytes. The circulating granulocyte turnover rate (GTR) also can be determined from the TBGP and the t$^{1/2}$ of granulocytes by the equation: GTR = 0.693/t$^{1/2}$ · TBGP

In summary, granulocytopoiesis consists of a fairly long bone marrow phase involving both proliferation and maturation and a very short period of circulation in peripheral blood. This is in contrast to erythroid cell kinetics in which the bone marrow proliferative phase is short and the life span of circulating red cells much longer. The rapid turnover of granulocytes in the circulation accounts for the 3:1 ratio of granulocyte precursors to erythroid precursors in bone marrow and the rapid development of granulocytopenia accompanying conditions in which marrow production of granulocytes is decreased.

9.2.9 REGULATION OF GRANULOCYTOPOIESIS

We do not have detailed knowledge of the factors controlling granulocytopoiesis. Humoral factors (granulopoietins) analogous to erythropoietin may be important in regulating the proliferation of granulocytic precursors. The precise nature of such substances is undetermined. Human urine and serum contain substances that can increase granulocytopoiesis in cell cultures, using semi-solid media. Peripheral WBC, used as a feeder layer in such cultures, produce a diffusible substance that is a potent stimulus for colony formation in this system. Evidence that this granulocyte colony-stimulating activity is equivalent to a physiologic granulopoietin is not available. Substances also have been isolated from granulocytes that inhibit granulocyte proliferation in vitro. These so-called granulocyte chalones may participate in the regulation of granulocytopoiesis. It is also possible that mature granulocytes exert negative feedback on granulocytopoiesis. Indirect evidence for this concept is derived from experiments that demonstrate that mixing mature granulocytes with more immature colony-forming granulocyte precursor cells inhibits colony formation.

ACTH and adrenal corticosteroids also induce granulocytopoiesis by accelerated release of bone marrow granulocytes, by a shift of granulocytes from the marginated to the circulating granulocyte pool and by inhibition of granulocyte migration from blood to tissues; it is doubtful whether these hormones are physiologic regulators of granulocytopoiesis. Epinephrine and exercise increase circulating granulocytes at the expense of the marginated granulocyte pool without a concomitant increase in marrow granulocyte proliferation.

9.2.10 GRANULOCYTOSIS ASSOCIATED WITH BENIGN DISORDERS

Infections are the most common cause of increased circulating granulocytes or *granu-*

locytosis. Tissue necrosis such as that accompanying myocardial infarction or hepatitis, metabolic disorders such as uremia and diabetic acidosis, burns, poisonings, stress and steroid therapy also are associated with granulocytosis. The granulocytosis in response to infection is primarily due to increased marrow granulocytopoiesis. In addition to an increase in the number of granulocytes in the peripheral blood, circulating immature forms (band forms, metamyelocytes and occasionally myelocytes) increase as well. The percentage of total WBC that are granulocytes increases from 60–70% to over 90%. These changes result from an increased outpouring of immature granulocytes from the bone marrow. Coarse basophilic granules called "toxic granules" may be found in granulocytes responding to infection. The clinical syndromes associated with benign or reactive granulocytoses, best exemplified by infection, vary with the specific etiology of the disorder. In bacterial infections the degree of fever, malaise and either local or systemic symptomatology depends on the specific organism and its pathogenicity. The total WBC count may range from just over 10,000 to as high as 60,000, although usually it is between 10,000 and 20,000.

When a reactive white count is over 30,000 and associated with circulating immature granulocytes, the leukocytosis is termed a *leukemoid reaction.* Severe leukemoid reactions are rare but may occur with acute infections, chronic infections such as tuberculosis, acute alcoholic hepatitis, burns, poisonings, cancer or lymphoma. The extreme leukocytosis and the immature granulocytes in a leukemoid reaction must be distinguished from the leukocytosis associated with myeloproliferative disorders, especially chronic myelogenous leukemia (CML). An increase of granulocytes in peripheral blood and of granulocyte precursors at all stages of maturation in bone marrow is characteristic of both severe reactive granulocytosis and CML. Leukemoid reactions usually disap-

pear with successful therapy of the underlying condition. In some cases, special clinical features such as the presence of splenomegaly, and special tests such as leukocyte alkaline phosphatase and karyotyping, may be necessary to distinguish between benign and malignant granulocytopoiesis; these will be discussed further in the section (11.5.1) on myeloproliferative disorders.

9.2.11 GRANULOCYTOPENIA AND ITS MECHANISMS

Decreased numbers of granulocytes in peripheral blood is termed *granulocytopenia.* *Agranulocytosis* describes a more severe form of this disorder (less than 300 granulocytes/cu mm). When patients have less than 1,000 granulocytes/cu mm, the risk of infection is significantly increased. Granulocytopenia can be due to decreased production, to increased destruction or to accelerated utilization of granulocytes. Specific mechanisms include:

1. Decreased production due to myelophthisis, i.e., replacement of marrow associated with cancer, leukemia, lymphoma or myelofibrosis.

2. Decreased production due to stem cell failure, as in aplastic anemia (see Chapter 3).

3. Decreased production or defective differentiation due to dietary deficiency, drugs, alcohol or infection. Malnutrition, folic acid and B_{12} deficiency and alcoholism are associated with granulocytopenia. Certain drugs occasionally cause neutropenia even in small doses. Chlorpromazine, for example, inhibits DNA synthesis in early neutrophilic precursors. Other drugs including many antileukemic agents, when given in sufficient amounts, consistently produce granulocytopenia by interfering with DNA synthesis and/or mitosis.

4. Increased destruction of granulocytes due to hypersplenism. Splenic sequestration of granulocytes due to splenomegaly of almost any etiology may lead to granulocytopenia. Infiltration of the spleen with lym-

phoma or leukemia, the Felty syndrome and congestive splenomegaly secondary to portal cirrhosis all can provide the anatomic basis for increased granulocytic sequestration.

5. Increased granulocyte destruction due to leukoagglutinins secondary to drugs such as aminopyrine and propylthiouracil. The destruction of agglutinated granulocytes occurs in the lungs as well as in other sites. Granulocyte precursors also may be affected and bone marrow examination will show the loss of myelocytes and myeloblasts.

6. Increased destruction due to leukocyte isoantibodies, especially following multiple blood transfusions and occasionally in SLE.

7. A variety of congenital disorders also are associated with either cyclic neutropenia or agranulocytosis, including infantile genetic agranulocytosis and familial neutropenia.

9.2.12 Clinical and Hematologic Manifestations of Granulocytopenia

Symptomatic granulocytopenia is characterized by malaise, sore throat, chills and fever. Oral mucus membrane ulceration is common. Careful history-taking may uncover potentially implicated drugs or toxic exposure. Splenomegaly on physical examination suggests hypersplenism, lymphoma or SLE. The blood count may show either isolated granulocytopenia or an associated thrombocytopenia or anemia as well. Examination of the bone marrow will reveal infiltrative disorders such as leukemia, lymphoma or cancer, aplastic anemia or myelofibrosis.

Most drug-related granulocytopenias are self-limited; the granulocyte count returns to normal after the drug is discontinued. The treatment of granulocytopenia when marrow disease exists is directed at the underlying disorder. In some instances of granulocytopenia associated with splenomegaly accompanied by severe recurrent infection, splenectomy may be indicated.

9.2.13 Eosinophils and Basophils

Elevated blood eosinophil levels (*eosinophilic granulocytosis* or *eosinophilia*) are characteristically seen in allergic states. Eosinophilia is seen accompanying (1) parasitic infiltrations, (2) hay fever and asthma, (3) drug hypersensitivity, (4) dermatologic disorders, (5) periarteritis nodosa and (6) pulmonary infiltrative disorders with eosinophilia (the Loeffler syndrome).

Basophilia in the peripheral blood is seen in CML, less often in other myeloproliferative disorders and some allergic reactions. Basophils are increased in delayed immune reactions, especially in local exudates accompanying these reactions.

9.2.14 Monocytosis

An increased number of monocytes accompanies a variety of hematologic and nonhematologic conditions including the myeloproliferative syndromes; lymphomas and other malignancies; and low grade infections, especially tuberculosis and subacute bacterial endocarditis.

9.3 Lymphocytes

9.3.1 Morphology

Lymphocytes are mononuclear cells with round or indented nuclei containing condensed chromatin (see Fig. 9–1). Nucleoli are absent. The cytoplasm is characteristically light blue and clear. A few azurophilic granules can be seen. Most lymphocytes are small (diameter about 10 mμ); however, there are variable numbers of larger lymphocytes seen in normal blood.

9.3.2 Origin and Function

Recent evidence indicates that lymphocytes are derived from stem cells in the bone marrow. Two lymphocyte populations can be differentiated: (1) those that originate in the bone marrow but are not exposed to the thymus, so-called B cells, responsible for antibody-mediated immunity; and (2) those that migrate to the thymus in the course of development, so-called thymus-derived or T cells, responsible for cell-mediated immune reactions. Both T and B lymphocytes migrate to lymph nodes and to the spleen where they proliferate and are stored. Lymphocytes circulate in the peripheral blood and recirculate through the blood, lymph nodes, spleen, thoracic duct and other tissues. The majority of circulating lymphocytes are long-lived cells (months to years) and are believed to be responsible for the immunologic competence of the host. A smaller population of short-lived lymphocytes also has been identified.

The major sites of storage of lymphocytes are the germinal centers of lymphoid follicles of the spleen and lymph nodes. Both lymphocyte proliferation and maturation are necessary for the immune response. The primary stimulus for proliferation of lymphocytes is exposure to antigens. B lymphocytes have the capacity to respond to a limited number of antigens by proliferating and by initiating synthesis of specific humoral antibody; T cells also participate in this reaction and are required for B lymphocytes to undergo an appropriate immunologic response. Antibodies also are formed by plasma cells that are derived from lymphocytes. T cells are considered to be active in the cellular immune response and delayed hypersensitivity. T cells are recognized by several criteria: (1) absence of antibody on their surface, (2) ability to form aggregates with sheep red blood cells (rosettes) and (3) presence of unique antigens on their surface. B cells are identified principally by the presence of surface Ig. In addition, B cells have surface receptors for certain components of the complement system and the Fc fragment of IgG.

9.3.3 RELATIONSHIP OF T AND B CELLS TO LYMPHOPROLIFERATIVE DISORDERS

Attempts are currently being made to demonstrate specific T and B cell dysfunction in disorders of the lymphoid system. In many cases of chronic lymphocytic leukemia (CLL), defective B cells having only small amounts of surface Ig are detected. Humoral immunity may be deficient in CLL, and B cell dysfunction may be implicated. In some lymphomas, especially Hodgkin's disease, cell-mediated immunity is diminished, suggesting a defect in the T cell system. In some cases of Hodgkin's disease and non-Hodgkin lymphoma, T cells comprise the major lymphoid cell type. However, other cases in which neither B or T cell markers can be identified have been described. Further definition of T and B cell populations and subpopulations in lymphoproliferative disorders may contribute to a more meaningful understanding of the underlying cellular and immunologic defects in these diseases.

9.3.4 LYMPHOCYTOSIS

Relative and absolute lymphocytosis may be observed in association with a spectrum of both benign and malignant disorders. Malignant lymphoproliferative disorders, including leukemia and the lymphomas, will be discussed subsequently (Chapter 12).

Lymphocytosis may occur during a number of acute infections, e.g., pertussis, acute infectious lymphocytosis and infectious mononucleosis, usually in children. In *infectious mononucleosis* abnormal lymphocytes in the blood smear will suggest the diagnosis, and determination of heterophil antibody titers will confirm it. The atypical lymphocytes of infectious mononucleosis are not pathognomonic for this disorder; they are observed in infectious hepatitis and other viral infections as well. In pertussis and acute infectious lymphocytosis, the number of lymphocytes may be markedly increased and morphologically indistinguishable from normal lymphocytes. Associated clinical and microbiologic features will lead to a correct diagnosis of these disorders. Thyrotoxicosis; toxoplasmosis; typhoid fever; brucellosis; viral infections such as measles, varicella, and cytomegalic inclusion disease and certain drug and allergic reactions may be associated with a relative increase in lymphocytes. However, the total lymphocyte count is usually below 20,000 in these disorders. In most disorders associated with benign lymphocytosis, bone marrow examination is normal or shows only a modest increase in lymphocytes. Relative marrow lymphocytosis also may accompany drug toxicity and is probably due to decreased production of granulocytic, erythroid and megakaryocytic precursors with preservation of lymphocytic cells.

10

Acute Leukemia

10.1 Introduction

THE ACUTE LEUKEMIAS are characterized by apparently uncontrolled proliferation of an abnormal population of immature hematopoietic cells, which may be lymphocytic, myelocytic or monocytic precursors. All of the acute leukemias have similar clinical and hematologic manifestations and they will be discussed together. Specific features characteristic of the several morphologic variants will be described as well.

10.2 Etiology

The precise mechanisms responsible for the unregulated emergence of a population of immature hematopoietic precursor cells in acute leukemia are unknown. Viruses are a proved cause of leukemia in experimental animals. Recent evidence strongly suggests that viruses may play a significant role in the etiology of acute leukemia in man but as yet there is no direct evidence for the viral etiology of human leukemia. There also are data that suggest that acute leukemia is due either to (1) the transformation of immature hematopoietic cells by exogenous viruses or other oncogenic agents, or (2) the activation of oncogenes (genes involved in malignant transformation) pre-existing in the involved cells. In either case, a population of cells emerges that fails to respond to the physiologic regulators that initiate differentiation and control proliferation in response to body needs. The presence of an RNA-dependent DNA polymerase (reverse transcriptase) has been detected in most oncogenic RNA viruses from animal species. This enzymatic activity also has been detected in human leukemic cells, providing circumstantial evidence for the presence of viral sequences in the development of human disease. In addition, it has been demonstrated that DNA sequences, present in human leukemic cells and absent from normal blood cells, show structural homology with RNA sequences from known murine leukemia viruses. Further studies will be necessary to determine whether viruses are truly etiologic agents in acute leukemia or merely associated with development of the disease. It also has been suggested that the accumulation of blast cells in acute leukemia is due to inhibition by viruses or other agents of the process of differentiation of otherwise normal blast cells. Observations that leukemic cells can differentiate to mature granulocytes in tissue culture are consistent with this hypothesis but require further documentation.

Ionizing radiation is one established factor in the development of acute leukemia as well as of chronic myelogenous leukemia (CML). There was an increased incidence of these leukemias (but not of chronic lymphocytic leukemia) among the survivors of the atomic bomb blasts in Hiroshima and Nagasaki and among patients receiving radiation for such conditions as ankylosing spondylitis. Industrial toxins, including chronic exposure to aromatic hydrocarbons, especially benzene, also have been associated with the development of acute leukemia. The development of acute leukemia in individuals exposed to irradiation and certain chemicals suggests that either (1) latent virus material present in cells may be activated by environmental changes, or (2) alterations in cellular DNA are induced by these agents, which predispose to leukemia.

Some cases of acute leukemia are preceded by an illness clinically indistinguishable from aplastic anemia. Rarely, aplastic anemia following the use of chloramphenicol and phenylbutazone has been followed by acute leukemia. More often, the syndrome of aplastic anemia that may precede acute leukemia is of unknown etiology.

In addition to these environmental factors, certain hereditary disorders are associated with the development of leukemia. There is a higher than normal incidence of acute leukemia in patients with the Down syndrome, the Bloom syndrome and Fanconi's anemia. There is no convincing evidence for an increased familial incidence of acute leukemia but there are case reports of the disease among siblings and relatives. There does appear to be a fourfold increased risk among siblings of leukemic children and a relatively high concordance of acute leukemia in monozygous twins. Although abnormalities of karyotype are seen in the blood cells of many patients with acute leukemia, there is no specific chromosomal pattern characteristic of these diseases, unlike that seen in CML (see section 11.5.1).

10.3 Pathogenesis

Regardless of the etiology, all acute leukemias are characterized by the presence of an abnormal hematopoietic cell population in the bone marrow of affected patients. Kinetic studies in most cases indicate that the abnormal precursor cells do not have significantly different cell cycle kinetics (mitotic index, labeling index or generation time) compared to normal cells at the same stage of differentiation. Thus, the acute leukemic cell in most cases is not proliferating at an abnormal rate; rather, it fails to differentiate normally and to cease proliferating, as a normal white cell precursor would do as it differentiates. The progeny of a normal myeloblast has differentiated and been destroyed within 10–14 days. By contrast, the malignant cells in acute leukemia fail to differentiate, accumulate in bone marrow and other tissues and eventually replace the normal hematopoietic elements, a process known as myelophthisis.

The blast cell population in acute leukemia is not homogeneous in its proliferative capacity. Labeling studies with tritiated thymidine indicate that only 30–50% of acute leukemia blast cells are actually in cell cycle, even as tested by a 24-hour exposure to ^{3}H-thymidine. This figure is not different from the percentage of normal myeloblasts in cell cycle. A rational therapy for acute leukemia must take into consideration this heterogeneity; leukemic cells are not uniformly susceptible to inhibitors of DNA synthesis or mitosis.

10.4 Clinical and Hematologic Findings

The increasing number of leukemic cells infiltrates bone marrow and may invade other organs as well, most commonly lymph nodes, liver and spleen, but the central nervous system and other nonhematopoietic sites also may be involved. The principal clinical manifestations result from a decrease in normal marrow elements. Decrease in erythroid precursors leads to anemia. Similarly, a decrease in the number of normal granulocytic precursors leads to granulocytopenia and an increased risk from infection. Decreased numbers of megakaryocytes lead to thrombocytopenia and predispose to bleeding. The triad of anemia, infection and bleeding represents a common manifestation of acute leukemia and comprises the major life-threatening manifestations of these disorders.

Acute leukemia may be either acute or insidious in onset. Symptoms consist primarily of weakness, malaise, lethargy, anorexia, fever, weight loss, pallor, bleeding and arthralgias. One or more of these symptoms usually cause the patient to seek medical care. The physical examination may be normal or there may be pallor, hemorrhagic manifestations, lymphadenopathy and hepa-

tosplenomegaly. Bone pain, especially sternal tenderness, due to marrow invasion is frequent particularly in children. Neurologic abnormalities associated with meningeal, cranial or peripheral nerve or root infiltration may be present.

Examination of the peripheral blood usually reveals anemia and thrombocytopenia. The WBC count is variable. It usually is increased due to the circulating leukemic cells (Fig. 10–1). However, the WBC count may be normal, and at times there may be few or no identifiable leukemic cells in the peripheral blood. Occasionally, the WBC count is below normal. When no leukemic cells are seen in the peripheral blood, the diagnosis of leukemia can be made or excluded only by bone marrow examination; this condition often is termed aleukemic leukemia.

10.5 Diagnosis

Diagnosis of acute leukemia depends on identifying an abnormal population of very immature hematopoietic precursor cells (usually more than 10%) in the bone marrow. The normal bone marrow contains less than 5% myeloblasts. The leukemic blast cells form a relatively homogeneous population of cells containing nucleoli and displaying variable but usually little evidence of cytologic

Fig. 10–1. – Blast cells in acute leukemia displaying high nucleo:cytoplasmic ratios and nucleoli.

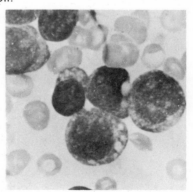

differentiation. In most cases the leukemic population represents the bulk of cells in the marrow. There is no increase in the intermediate and maturing granulocytic precursors, as is found in the benign reactive granulocytoses (see section 9.2.10) or in CML (see section 11.5). There is no specific diagnostic test for acute leukemia; a blast cell population in the marrow, together with anemia and thrombocytopenia, provides the most reliable diagnostic criterion. Infectious mononucleosis, maturation arrest in the granulocyte series secondary to drugs, infectious disorders associated with lymphocytosis and aplastic anemia must be considered in the differential diagnosis.

Two major types of acute leukemia are distinguished: acute lymphocytic (or lymphoblastic) leukemia (ALL) and acute granulocytic (or myelogenous) leukemia (AML).

10.5.1 ACUTE LYMPHOCYTIC LEUKEMIA

ALL is primarily a disease of children. The predominant cell in the bone marrow is a lymphoblast, an immature lymphocytoid cell containing nucleoli and somewhat clumped chromatin (see Fig. 10–1). Scant cytoplasm containing few, if any, granules is typical. Two populations of lymphoblasts may be distinguished in some patients: large lymphoblasts (which may be the most actively proliferating cells) and a class of smaller lymphoblasts. The significance of the two populations is unclear. Lymphoblasts do not stain with myeloperoxidase or lipid stains and contain little, if any, lysozyme. Lysozyme is an enzyme present in largest amounts in monocytes, present in significant amounts in granulocytes and absent in lymphocytes. In ALL, the serum lysozyme level usually is markedly decreased, whereas in granulocytic or monocytic leukemia the lysozyme level may be either normal or increased. ALL in children is the most responsive of the acute leukemias to therapy.

Between 25% and 50% of patients treated intensively with current chemotherapy regimens (see section 10.7.4) and prophylactic x-irradiation of the central nervous system (see section 10.7.3) survive more than 5 years.

10.5.2 ACUTE MYELOGENOUS (MYELOBLASTIC, GRANULOCYTIC) LEUKEMIA

AML is a disease primarily of adults, although it affects children as well. The malignant cell is a myeloblast that may resemble the normal myeloblast; it has a fine chromatin pattern, prominent, usually multiple, nucleoli and scant basophilic cytoplasm. Some cytoplasmic granules may be present and a modest degree of granulocytic differentiation sometimes may be detected by the myeloperoxidase stain. Characteristic eosinophilic cytoplasmic inclusions known as Auer rods may be found in leukemic myeloblasts. These structures appear to represent defective or arrested granule formation. The presence of Auer rods strongly supports the diagnosis of AML, although they also are found in some cases of myelomonocytic and monocytic leukemia. An increased number of promyelocytes as well as myeloblasts in occasional patients with AML is another manifestation of abortive differentiation of the leukemic cell line. The normal orderly progression of granulocytic maturation is, however, characteristically absent in AML. The serum lysozyme is usually normal or elevated.

The clinical presentation of AML is similar to that of ALL. Symptoms and signs due to anemia, infection and bleeding are the major manifestations. The prognosis in AML, whether in children or adults, is extremely poor. Approximately 50% of patients attain chemotherapy-induced remissions, but the duration of remission is usually less than 1 year (see section 10.7.5). Patients with AML, as well as with ALL, succumb either to uncontrolled bleeding, to infection due to the progression of disease or to the cytotoxic effects of therapy.

10.5.3 UNCOMMON TYPES OF ACUTE LEUKEMIA

These include (1) acute myelomonocytic leukemia, (2) acute monocytic leukemia, (3) acute promyelocytic leukemia and (4) the erythroleukemias. *Acute myelomonocytic leukemia* (Naegli type) is considered to reflect the neoplastic transformation of a stem cell, which displays limited differentiation along both the myeloblastic and monocytic pathways. In *acute monocytic leukemia* (Schilling type), the leukemic cell closely resembles an immature monocyte and has a lobulated nucleus. In both these forms of acute leukemia, the urinary lysozyme content usually is markedly elevated. In *acute promyelocytic leukemia* the predominant cell is the promyelocyte. This disorder may be associated with the syndrome of disseminated intravascular coagulation (DIC).

The *erythroleukemias* are characterized by a malignant hematopoietic proliferation predominantly of erythroid and myeloid precursors. There are both acute and chronic forms of the disease (also known as the Di Guglielmo syndrome). In the erythroleukemias there is either a rapid or insidious evolution of a population of bizarre erythroid precursors in bone marrow and occasionally in peripheral blood associated with a clinical picture resembling AML. The abnormal cells include macronormoblasts, cells with abnormal nuclear chromatin configuration and increased and atypical mitotic figures. This disorder must be distinguished from the megaloblastic anemias associated with vitamin B_{12} or folate deficiency, which also can be accompanied by pancytopenia. In the more acute form the erythroleukemic phase is temporary and often terminates in typical AML.

In each of these variants of acute leukemia, the clinical symptomatology is related to the presence of the abnormal population of cells and the deficiency of normal marrow elements, leading to thrombocytopenia, granulocytopenia and anemia. The course and prognosis are similar to those of patients with AML. Therapy is with the same agents used in other forms of acute leukemia (see section 10.7.2). Remissions are infrequent and of short duration, usually measured in months.

10.6 Differential Diagnosis

Since there is no single definitive test for the diagnosis of acute leukemia, it is essential to distinguish and exclude benign conditions that may mimic acute leukemia. For example, ALL in children can be confused with infectious lymphocytosis, reactive lymphocytosis due to pertussis or chronic infections, and infectious mononucleosis. The clinical symptoms of acute leukemia and infectious mononucleosis may at times be similar.

As in acute leukemia, infectious mononucleosis may present with fever, malaise and weakness, and the physical examination may reveal lymphadenopathy, splenomegaly and hepatomegaly. Pharyngitis and skin rash, relatively rare in acute leukemia, are common in infectious mononucleosis. Thrombocytopenia and anemia are quite rare in infectious mononucleosis but common in acute leukemia; their presence dictates an investigation for leukemia. Laboratory studies in infectious mononucleosis usually will show a normal or moderately elevated WBC and a normal platelet count; the circulating white cells show an increase in mononuclear cells including monocytes, lymphocytes and so-called atypical lymphocytes. These large and pleomorphic cells also are present in other viral diseases. They often contain abundant cytoplasm that is deep blue or foamy and vacuolated. The bone marrow in infectious mononucleosis is usually normal, with no abnormal blast cell population. In addition, a positive Paul-Bunnell test (heterophil agglutinins absorbable by beef erythrocyte antigen and not by guinea pig kidney) and the presence of antibody to Epstein-Barr virus confirm the diagnosis of infectious mononucleosis.

Pancytopenia due to aplastic anemia (see Chapter 3), megaloblastic anemia (see Chapter 5), or nonleukemic myelophthisis initially may suggest the diagnosis of acute leukemia; however, evaluation of the bone marrow will establish the proper diagnosis. In this regard, if no cells are obtained by needle aspiration ("dry tap"), a bone marrow biopsy should be performed, since in acute leukemia and other infiltrative conditions, invasive cells may pack the marrow so tightly as to preclude aspiration of its cellular content.

10.7 Therapy

Therapy falls into two general categories: (1) supportive and (2) specific chemotherapy.

10.7.1 SUPPORTIVE THERAPY

The goals of supportive therapy include:

1. *Control of bleeding.* If thrombocytopenia is severe (less than 10,000) or if bleeding occurs at any low platelet count, platelet transfusions are given. (Platelets can be obtained as fresh concentrates at major blood centers.) A rise in the platelet count following platelet transfusion is expected. However, even in the absence of an increase in platelet number, use of the infused platelets may forestall hemorrhagic complications. Although platelet transfusions are not usually HL-A typed, platelets do contain HL-A antigens, and antibodies to platelets often appear after several platelet transfusions. Prednisone in doses of 30–40 mg/day also can help reduce the danger of hemorrhage, presumably by an effect on vascular fragility. In patients with over 100,000 blasts/cu mm in peripheral blood, the risk from cerebral hemorrhage due to vascular lesions and infiltrates is high. This should be considered a medical emergency, and rapid initiation of specific chemotherapy is indicated.

2. *Control of anemia.* Blood transfusion should be provided if anemia is severe and symptomatic, or if there is significant hemorrhage.

3. *Prevention of uric acid nephropathy.* The proliferation of a large leukemic cell population can be associated with excessive accumulation of the products of cellular catabolism. Particularly ominous is hyperuricemia. When treatment with specific chemotherapy is begun, the incremental lysis of a large number of blasts results in a further increase in nucleic acid breakdown. Large amounts of additional uric acid are generated and may induce severe hyperuricemia and uric acid nephropathy. Uric acid is deposited in the renal collecting system and distal tubules and may result in acute renal failure. Allopurinol, a xanthine oxidase inhibitor, blocks conversion of relatively soluble xanthine to relatively insoluble uric acid and is the drug of choice for preventing hyperuricemia. Adequate hydration also is important in preventing uric acid nephropathy.

4. *Control of infections.* The most common cause of death in patients with acute leukemia is uncontrolled infection. Although low grade fever may be due to the disease alone, the threat of bacterial infection is severe, and appropriate cultures must always be taken. If a pathogenic organism is identified, specific antimicrobial treatment should begin before chemotherapy is started. When patients already have been treated with chemotherapy or are severely granulocytopenic because of the leukemia, infection is particularly ominous and must be treated promptly and vigorously. Under these conditions, when a significant fever spike (usually greater than 102 F) occurs, cultures are obtained and the patient placed on a combination of antibiotics effective against both gram-positive and gram-negative bacteria. The most frequent pathogens are Pseudomonas, Proteus, *Escherichia coli* and staphylococcus. A cephalosporin and gentamicin and/or carbenicillin are most frequently used.

Leukemic patients are very susceptible to opportunistic infections. The possibility of a fungal infection must be evaluated by appropriate cultures; systemic mycosis is currently treated with amphotericin. Other opportunistic infections that must be considered in patients with acute leukemia include those caused by *Pneumocystis carinii,* toxoplasmosis and cytomegalic inclusion virus disease. The most frequent site of infection is the lungs; lung biopsy may be necessary to establish an early and definitive diagnosis. Perirectal abscesses and urinary tract and meningeal infections also may be encountered.

10.7.2 Specific Chemotherapy

The goal of specific chemotherapy is to eradicate the leukemic cell population and to spare normal bone marrow precursor cells. Agents that would selectively attack leukemic cells would be highly desirable but do not exist. A partial exception to this is L-asparaginase, an enzyme available for clinical use. L-Asparaginase preferentially kills cells that require an exogenous supply of the amino acid, asparagine. Most normal cells do not require this amino acid, whereas certain leukemic cells do. However, in clinical practice, L-asparaginase used alone is of only limited value because of the emergence of leukemic cell variants or mutants that are resistant to the effects of the enzyme.

As discussed previously, the leukemic cell population contains cells in two functional states: (1) cells in cell cycle, and (2) resting cells not in cell cycle. The therapeutic attack must be designed to deal with both. The majority of currently available chemotherapeutic agents (Table 10–1) are effective because of their inhibitory effects on DNA synthesis or mitosis (cell cycle-active agents). 6-Mercaptopurine, 6-thioguanine, daunomycin and methotrexate all act on cells by inhibiting DNA synthesis, although at different sites in the DNA biosynthetic pathway. The vinca alkaloids, vincristine and vinblastine, are effective against cells that enter mitosis and perhaps on resting cells as well. When cell cycle-active agents are given to patients with acute leukemia, those leukemic cells in cell cycle are rapidly destroyed. Unavoidably, normal marrow precursor cells of the erythroid, myeloid and megakaryocytic series that are proliferating also are affected by the cytotoxic agents. The reason for the effectiveness of cell cycle-active agents has not yet been fully explained. The apparently successful eradication of all acute leukemic cells in "cured" children with ALL, for example, whereas normal stem cells are at least partially spared, suggests (1) that there may be a differential susceptibility of leukemic cells to chemotherapeutic agents, (2) that more normal stem cells than leukemic cells may be out of cell cycle or (3) that, after most leukemic cells have been killed, host immune mechanisms can eradicate the remaining leukemic cell population.

It is also necessary to eradicate leukemic cells that are nonproliferating (resting, not in cell cycle). Relatively few agents are effective in this regard. These drugs include the adrenocortical steroids, the nitrosoureas and other alkylating agents. Steroids have a pronounced lymphocytolytic effect but their precise mechanism of action is unknown. Alkylating agents and the nitrosoureas are effective since they alter proteins and nucleic acids in both resting and replicating cells. A potentially useful characteristic of acute leukemic cells is that, as the number of cells in cell cycle is reduced by therapy, more resting cells enter cell cycle and become susceptible to cell cycle-active agents. This recruitment of resting cells into cycle appears to play an important role in the success of therapy with cell cycle-active agents. Thus, the continued administration of cell cycle-active agents has proved to be the most effective way of reducing the leukemic cell population.

The successful use of combinations of antibiotics in certain bacterial infections to prevent the rapid emergence of resistant organisms has been adapted to the treatment of

TABLE 10-1.—AGENTS IN TREATMENT OF LEUKEMIA

AGENT	MECHANISM OF ACTION	CLINICAL EFFICACY*	TOXIC SIDE EFFECTS†
Prednisone	Lympholytic	ALL, CLL	Hypertension, diabetes, osteoporosis, psychoses, peptic ulcer
Vincristine	Inhibitor of mitosis	ALL, AML	Alopecia, neurotoxicity (esp. peripheral neuropathy), ileus
6-Mercaptopurine	Purine antagonist, inhibits DNA synthesis	ALL, AML	Nausea, vomiting, hepatotoxicity
Methotrexate	Folic acid antagonist; inhibits DNA synthesis	ALL, AML	Oral and gastrointestinal ulceration, hepatotoxicity
Daunomycin	Intercalates in DNA; inhibits DNA replication	ALL, AML	Cardiac failure, alopecia
Cytosine arabinoside	Pyrimidine analog; inhibits DNA synthesis	AML	Nausea, vomiting, megaloblastic anemia
6-Thioguanine	Purine antagonist; inhibits DNA synthesis	ALL, AML	Nausea, vomiting, hepatotoxicity
Nitrosourea (BCNU, CCNU‡)	Alkylating agents; inhibit DNA and protein synthesis	AML	Nausea, vomiting
Cyclophosphamide	Alkylating agent; inhibits DNA and protein synthesis	AML	Hemorrhagic cystitis, hepatotoxicity
Busulfan	Alkylating agent; inhibits DNA and protein synthesis	CML	Pulmonary fibrosis, skin pigmentation
Chlorambucil	Alkylating agent; inhibits DNA and protein synthesis	CLL	Hepatotoxicity
Hydroxyurea	Inhibits DNA synthesis	AML, ALL, CML	
L-Asparaginase	Destroys asparagine	ALL	Allergic reactions, coagulopathy, hepatotoxicity, pancreatitis

*ALL = acute lymphocytic leukemia; CLL = chronic lymphocytic leukemia; AML = acute myelogenous leukemia; CML = chronic myelogenous leukemia.
†All agents in significant doses lead to bone marrow hypoplasia.
‡BCNU = 1, 3-bis(2-chloroethyl)-1-nitrosourea; CCNU = 1-(2-chloroethyl)-3-cyclohexyl-1-nitrosurea.

acute leukemia. Combinations of drugs with different mechanisms of action have been shown to prevent the proliferation and survival of leukemic cells resistant to any single drug, and this combination chemotherapy is superior to single-agent treatment in the induction of remission in leukemia. Complete remission is achieved when there is no evidence in the peripheral blood and bone marrow of leukemia. Usually, in order to achieve complete remission, it is necessary to induce profound bone marrow hypoplasia and pancytopenia. Subsequently, in patients who respond to chemotherapy, normal marrow elements return, whereas leukemic cells do not, for the duration of the remission.

It has become apparent, however, that in remission, although bone marrow reveals no identifiable leukemic cells, there still may be significant numbers of leukemic cells in the marrow or elsewhere, too few to recognize but enough to initiate relapse unless chemotherapy is continued. As many as 10^9 leukemic cells distributed throughout the total bone marrow can elude detection by marrow examination. For these reasons, another principle of chemotherapy is "consolidation", i.e., intensive treatment with chemotherapeutic agents following induction of complete remission in an attempt to kill the remaining leukemic cells that cannot be seen on bone marrow smear. This therapy also is directed at leukemic cells that were not in cell cycle during induction therapy but that may be recruited into cell cycle subsequently. Following consolidation, less intensive "maintenance" chemotherapy is provided, with the goal of continued eradication of residual leukemic cells and prolongation of the remission.

10.7.3 EXTRAMEDULLARY LEUKEMIC INFILTRATES

These pose another threat to the leukemic patient. Although the bone marrow may be completely cleared of leukemic cells, certain tissues such as the central nervous system and testes, with their unique vascular supply, are not readily accessible to systemic chemotherapy and may contain significant numbers of residual leukemic cells despite marrow and blood remission. The prophylactic use of cranial irradiation and intrathecal drugs has significantly decreased the incidence of central nervous system relapse in leukemic patients.

10.7.4 CHEMOTHERAPY IN ALL

Since no completely effective therapy is yet available, optimal chemotherapeutic regimens in the treatment of acute leukemia are constantly changing. The treatment program that follows is an example of one current regimen. Although it exemplifies the principles of leukemia therapy discussed earlier, the specific drugs used and their schedule of administration undoubtedly will change with further experience.

Vincristine and steroids in combination have been shown to induce a remission in approximately 90% of children with ALL. Following remission, a course of L-asparaginase may be given. This is followed by 6-mercaptopurine and methotrexate given either parenterally or by mouth for approximately 2 years. In addition, the combination of cranial radiotherapy and intrathecal methotrexate therapy is used prophylactically for residual central nervous system disease. With these intensive therapeutic programs, the current prognosis in childhood ALL anticipates that 25–50% of children will be in complete remission after 5 years, with normal bone marrow and peripheral blood findings. It should be noted, however, that a relapse at any time after initial therapy markedly reduces the probability for long-term survival and possible cure.

In ALL in adults the same drugs and treatment programs are used as in children. The remission rate in adults, however, is only 50–70%, and the average duration of remission is only 1 year.

10.7.5 CHEMOTHERAPY IN AML

Cytosine arabinoside, thioguanine and daunomycin are presently the most effective drugs for inducing remission in AML; a remission rate of 40–50% can be expected with these drugs used in combination. However, as yet no really adequate consolidation or maintenance chemotherapy has been found that will produce the prolonged remissions seen in childhood ALL. The average duration of remission for patients with AML who respond to therapy is only 11 months, whereas patients who fail to achieve a remission with chemotherapy usually die within 3 months. The design and testing of newer regimens for the induction and maintenance of remissions in AML remain a most challenging problem in leukemia research.

10.8 Newer Therapeutic Approaches

10.8.1 IMMUNOTHERAPY

The proposed use of immunotherapy in acute leukemia is based on observations that suggest that leukemic cells contain unique surface antigens that distinguish them from normal cells. It has been postulated that defective immunologic surveillance permits uncontrolled proliferation of leukemic cells in susceptible patients. The goal of immunotherapy is to stimulate host immune responses to destroy the leukemic cells. In experimental animals it has been found that immunologic stimulants are most effective when the number of tumor cells is small. Thus, these agents are being tested principally in patients who have achieved complete clinical remission on chemotherapy. BCG has been reported to prolong remission duration in ALL, but other studies have yet to confirm this observation. BCG, as well as other nonspecific stimulators of the reticuloendothelial system of macrophages such as MER (a methanol extractable residue of BCG), and *carini bacterium parvum,* a nonpathogenic bacterial preparation, are presently undergoing clinical trials. Poly I:C, a polyinosinic-polycytidylic acid synthetic polynucleotide, an inducer of interferon, is likewise being tested for clinical effectiveness. The identification of specific leukemia cell antigens and immunization of leukemic patients with these antigens represent another area of current clinical investigation.

10.8.2 BONE MARROW TRANSPLANTATION

With growing understanding of the genetic histocompatibility loci in man, the use of normal bone marrow transplantation after treatment with chemotherapy has been attempted in patients with acute leukemia. Successful bone marrow transplants from identical twins and from histocompatible siblings have been reported. Marrow transplantation, at present, must be considered an experimental therapy requiring a major institutional commitment of staff and facilities including histocompatibility typing, provision of supportive blood products (platelets and granulocytes), isolation and bacteriologic support services and an experienced clinical transplantation team. Successful transplantation at present requires preliminary antileukemia chemotherapy, as well as intensive immunosuppression and total body x-irradiation, for recipients of matched but not syngeneic (identical twin) donor marrow. In most patients in whom transplantation has been successfully accomplished, leukemic cells have ultimately re-emerged with a fatal outcome. In two cases it has been reported that the recurring leukemic cell population may have been derived from the marrow donor as determined by karyotype, suggesting an infectious agent or other leukemogenic factor in the recipient. In the majority of cases, recrudescence of leukemia appears to be due to residual leukemic cells in the marrow recipient.

10.8.3 GERM-FREE ENVIRONMENTS AND GRANULOCYTE TRANSFUSIONS

Measures for prevention of infections include the use of (1) isolation units with filtered laminar air flow to protect patients from exogenous pathogens, (2) granulocyte transfusions for granulocytopenia and (3) prophylactic nonabsorbable oral antibiotics to reduce intestinal bacterial flora. Utilization of these measures separately and in combination is currently under evaluation. At present, the use of granulocyte transfusions is limited because of their short functional half-life, although encouraging reports of reduced morbidity and mortality due to sepsis in leukopenic subjects receiving granulocyte infusions are accumulating.

11

Myeloproliferative Syndromes

11.1 Introduction

THE MYELOPROLIFERATIVE SYNDROMES constitute a group of disorders discussed together because of certain common features; they include polycythemia vera, myeloid metaplasia, chronic myelogenous leukemia (CML) and acute myelogenous leukemia (AML; see Chapter 10). These disorders are interrelated because of what clinically appears to be occasional or regular transitions from one syndrome to another. For example, polycythemia vera may progress to myeloid metaplasia, and myeloid metaplasia may terminate in acute leukemia. Each of these disorders has in common the proliferation of one or more marrow elements. In polycythemia vera erythroid, myeloid and megakaryocytic precursors are increased, presumably due to an abnormality in a common hematopoietic stem cell. In myeloid metaplasia associated with myelofibrosis, fibroblast proliferation in the marrow is characteristic. In CML the entire spectrum of granulocytic cells is increased; in AML an abnormal population of differentiation-defective early granulocyte precursors is implicated (see section 10.5.2).

11.2 Polycythemia Vera

Polycythemia vera is a disease of adults characterized by erythremia and variable degrees of leukocytosis and thrombocytosis. In most cases increased red cell production is the predominant feature. In the majority of cases also, some degree of thrombocytosis and leukocytosis occurs during the course of the disease. Symptoms, if present, usually reflect hyperviscosity of the blood, sluggish blood flow and a propensity to thrombosis. These symptoms include tinnitus, headache, pruritus, dizziness, epigastric distress, peptic ulcer disease, gastrointestinal bleeding, angina pectoris and cerebrovascular insufficiency. On physical examination, splenomegaly is frequent, and hepatomegaly also may occur. Hyperuricemia is present in the majority of patients. The hemoglobin level is often greater than 17 gm/100 ml but may be only slightly elevated. The WBC count usually is greater than 12,000/cu mm and the platelet count is commonly elevated as well. There is no single diagnostic test that establishes the diagnosis of polycythemia vera; combined elevation of RBC, WBC and platelet counts is highly suggestive, but other conditions causing erythremia must be ruled out. These include the following:

1. *Erythremia secondary to cardiopulmonary disease,* which produces arterial oxygen unsaturation; this condition can be distinguished by appropriate blood gas and cardiopulmonary studies.

2. *Erythremia occasionally associated with renal disorders and renal, uterine, hepatic and cerebellar tumors;* inappropriate production of erythropoietin sometimes can be demonstrated.

3. *Rare abnormal hemoglobins* with increased oxygen affinity such as the Chesapeake, Yakima and Takoma hemoglobins; these usually can be diagnosed by hemoglobin electrophoresis and by an abnormal oxygen dissociation curve (see section 8.6.2). Some high oxygen-affinity hemoglobins have been reported with no electrophoretic abnormality; these require special tests for their detection.

4. *Relative erythremia* due solely to a decrease in plasma volume, with no increase in absolute red cell mass. This condition can be established by measurements of red cell and plasma volume with ^{51}Cr-labeled red cells and ^{131}I-labeled albumin, respectively.

When the diagnosis of polycythemia vera is confirmed, therapy is directed at the most serious clinical problems. If erythremia predominates, phlebotomy is the treatment of choice and can rapidly ameliorate symptoms of hyperviscosity. Regular phlebotomy can be used for many years to control erythremia. When thrombocytosis is the most severe problem, intermittent busulfan, an alkylating agent, has proved effective. Radioactive phosphorus (^{32}P) also is an effective form of therapy for polycythemia vera and can control both erythremia and thrombocytosis. However, the possibility of an increased incidence of acute leukemia in patients treated with ^{32}P has generated some reappraisal of this modality. The relative merits of phlebotomy and ^{32}P have yet to be fully resolved. The erythremia and thrombocytosis of polycythemia vera should be treated because they entail increased risk of bleeding and thrombosis. Peptic ulcer disease, severe complications associated with surgery and hyperviscosity syndromes are all common in poorly controlled patients.

11.3 Essential Thrombocythemia

In this disorder thrombocytosis predominates, whereas leukocytosis and erythremia are minimal or absent. Splenomegaly is present early in the course of this disease in the majority of patients. The patient is exposed to an increased risk of thrombotic and hemorrhagic complications. Busulfan has been effective in reducing dangerously elevated platelet counts.

11.4 Myeloid Metaplasia with Myelofibrosis

Myeloid metaplasia with myelofibrosis (also called agnogenic myeloid metaplasia) is a disorder of unknown etiology in which the bone marrow is fibrotic and there is extramedullary hematopoiesis in the liver, spleen and less commonly other sites such as lymph nodes. The temporal or etiologic relationship between the development of myelofibrosis in the marrow and the proliferation of hematopoietic elements in extramedullary sites is unclear.

11.4.1 CLINICAL PATTERN

The disorder is associated with fatigue, pallor, weight loss and anorexia and hepatosplenomegaly on physical examination. Abdominal discomfort due to splenomegaly is common. Examination of the peripheral blood usually reveals leukocytosis together with immature granulocytes including myelocytes and occasionally myeloblasts in the peripheral blood; WBC counts may reach 40,000/cu mm. Careful evaluation of the peripheral smear can contribute significantly to a correct diagnosis. Typical findings include abnormal red cell morphology with many tear-drop forms, anisocytosis, poikilocytosis and the presence of nucleated red cells (see section 2.6). In addition to red cell changes and the presence of immature granulocytic cells, giant platelets and platelet aggregates are often seen. These peripheral blood findings are characteristic and strongly suggest the diagnosis, although they may be observed in other causes of myelophthisis such as metastatic tumor or granulomatous disease. Anemia is usually present and results from decreased bone marrow erythropoiesis, hypersplenism, folic acid deficiency, bleeding or a combination of these mechanisms.

11.4.2 Diagnosis

A bone marrow biopsy demonstrating myelofibrosis is the definitive diagnostic test. Bone marrow aspiration is usually unsuccessful and of little or no help since any cause of myelophthisis or aplastic anemia may result in a "dry tap." Myeloid metaplasia with myelofibrosis must be distinguished from acute leukemia, aplastic anemia and CML. Therapy is unsatisfactory in most cases and consists of transfusions, folic acid and androgens for treatment of anemia; busulfan, splenectomy or splenic irradiation has been used to treat symptomatic hypersplenism or splenic discomfort. Splenectomy may be counterproductive when the spleen is the major site of hematopoiesis. Massive splenomegaly, thrombocytopenia, anemia and the development of acute leukemia are all complications of this disorder, although some patients survive with their disease for many years.

11.5 Chronic Myelogenous (Myelocytic or Granulocytic) Leukemia

CML is a malignant disorder of hematopoiesis characterized by increased numbers of granulocytic cells at all stages of maturation, both proliferating in the bone marrow and circulating in the peripheral blood. Onset of the disease is often insidious. Symptoms include fatigue and weakness, less often fever and night sweats. Physical examination usually reveals marked splenomegaly by the time the diagnosis is recognized and may demonstrate hepatomegaly as well. Peripheral blood counts show a marked leukocytosis with WBC counts greater than 20,000 and often over 100,000/cu mm. Many immature granulocytic forms are present including metamyelocytes, myelocytes and occasionally promyelocytes and blasts as well. Increased numbers of eosinophils and basophils are regularly seen. Mild anemia may be present, and thrombocytosis, often above one million/cu mm, may be manifest early in the course of the disease. Bone marrow examination shows a predominance of granulocytic cells (an increased myeloid:erythroid ratio) and a shift toward immature forms. Unlike acute leukemia, there is no predominant population of blast cells. Information obtained by history, physical examination and evaluation of peripheral blood and bone marrow findings may not always be sufficient to distinguish between a diagnosis of CML and diseases associated with a benign or reactive leukemoid reaction (see section 9.2.10).

11.5.1 Diagnosis

Differentiation of CML from leukemoid reactions can be aided by the demonstration of (1) the Ph[1] chromosome, and (2) decreased leukocyte alkaline phosphatase (LAP) level.

The *Ph[1] chromosome,* an abnormal chromosome 22 lacking a portion of its longer arm, is present in the myeloid cells of more than 80% of patients with CML. Although the precise significance of the Ph¹ chromosome is unknown, it is the only specific chromosomal abnormality so far identified in a malignant disease; it is not seen in reactive leukocytosis. The Ph¹ chromosome also is present in erythroid and megakaryocytic precursor cells but not in nonhematopoietic cells. This is consistent with the evidence that a single bone marrow stem cell differentiates into erythroid, granulocytic and megakaryocytic cell lines (see section 1.5). The Ph¹ chromosome is not found in the cells of identical twins of patients with CML, which suggests that it is an acquired alteration in the hematopoietic stem cell. In females heterozygous for type A and B variants of the X chromosome-linked enzyme, G-6-PD, all cells that contain the Ph¹ chromosome contain the same isoenzyme, either A or B, but not both. This strongly supports the hypothesis that malignant transformation occurs in a single hematopoietic stem cell, producing a growing clone of leukemic cells.

Leukocyte alkaline phosphatase is an enzyme normally present in mature granulocytes that can be quantitated by a cytochemical stain. The amount of stainable LAP is usually markedly diminished or absent in the mature granulocytes of patients with CML, whereas it is normal or elevated in those with leukemoid reactions and polycythemia vera. Decreased LAP staining also may be observed in paroxysmal nocturnal hemoglobinuria (see section 6.8).

11.5.2 THERAPY AND COURSE

In most patients with CML, busulfan is effective in controlling the granulocyte count, decreasing spleen size, correcting anemia and thrombocytosis and improving the sense of well-being. Eventually, after an average remission duration of 36–40 months, most patients with CML become refractory to chemotherapy. Most often the disease terminates by transformation to a clinical picture virtually indistinguishable from AML, termed "blast crisis." Anemia, thrombocytopenia and emergence of a population of myeloblasts are characteristic. The blast crisis of CML is extremely resistant to chemotherapy and usually is fatal within 3 months. In patients with previously unrecognized CML who are seen initially in blast crisis, demonstration of the Ph¹ chromosome indicates the presence of antecedent CML. Patients with Ph¹-negative CML tend to be more resistant to busulfan therapy from the start. They usually have a shorter interval preceding blast crisis and an average life span of less than 10 months from the time of diagnosis.

12

Lymphoproliferative Diseases

12.1 Chronic Lymphocytic Leukemia

CLL IS A SLOWLY PROGRESSIVE lymphoproliferative disorder of the elderly involving predominantly the small lymphocytes. The abnormal cells are found in large numbers in the circulation, and they may infiltrate marrow, lymph nodes, spleen, liver and other organs as well. In this latter respect, CLL can be pathologically indistinguishable from well-differentiated lymphocytic lymphoma.

12.1.1 ETIOLOGY AND PATHOGENESIS

The etiology of CLL is unknown. The abnormal lymphocytes in many, but not all, cases studied appear to be defective B cells with small amounts of immunoglobulin (Ig) on their surface. Defective Ig production and

associated hypogammaglobulinemia are often a component of this disease. CLL lymphocytes also demonstrate abnormal delayed hypersensitivity responses and deficient blastogenic response to mitogen stimulation. Kinetic studies indicate that the immunologically incompetent CLL lymphocytes have an unusually long life span, accounting perhaps for the insidious and progressive accumulation of this cell population in the course of the disease. It is possible that CLL is a disorder of lymphocyte differentiation.

12.1.2 CLINICAL AND HEMATOLOGIC FINDINGS

Many patients with CLL are asymptomatic at the time of diagnosis, the disorder being discovered on routine blood count or because of asymptomatic lymphadenopathy. Others complain of fatigue, malaise and weight loss. Some degree of lymphadenopathy and hepatosplenomegaly is usually present at the time of diagnosis but these may develop gradually as the disease progresses. Blood count usually reveals a markedly elevated WBC count, often exceeding 100,000/cu mm; the majority of the cells are mature-appearing small lymphocytes. Small numbers of more immature lymphocytes are not uncommon. The diagnosis may be suspected but not proved in an older patient with a persistent modest lymphocytosis, if other causes are excluded. The development of frank CLL may take several years, attesting to its relatively indolent progression. Anemia and thrombocytopenia are uncommon in the majority of patients until later stages of the disease. Bone marrow examination shows a predominance of small lymphocytes; there is nothing pathognomonic about this infiltration and a bone marrow examination is not required to make the diagnosis.

If organ infiltration is the predominant manifestation, CLL may be difficult to distinguish from lymphocytic lymphoma and lymphosarcoma cell leukemia. In this latter disorder, lymphocytic infiltrates in lymph nodes and other organs are associated with lymphosarcoma cell lymphocytosis in bone marrow and peripheral blood. Lymphosarcoma cells are immature nucleolated lymphocytes with characteristic indentations of the nucleus. In these cases a diagnosis of either lymphosarcoma cell leukemia or lymphoproliferative disease with CLL is reasonable.

12.1.3 COURSE AND PROGNOSIS

The course and prognosis in CLL are better than in most hematologic malignancies. The duration of life from time of diagnosis averages 6–8 years. Prolonged survival (over 10 years) is not at all uncommon. The course of CLL is related to the progression of defective immunologic functions and to the extent of infiltration of normal hematopoietic tissues. The major immunologic defect in CLL is hypogammaglobulinemia and deficient humoral antibody production. The result is an increased frequency of infection.

Paradoxically, CLL is associated on occasion with inappropriate Ig production, most notably autoimmune hemolytic anemia (Coombs-positive anemia); more rarely, autoimmune thrombocytopenia and monoclonal dysproteinemia occur. Death from CLL is often related to infection or to marrow failure, with gradual extension of the lymphocytic disease, which becomes refractory to chemotherapy. The cumulative myelosuppressive and immunosuppressive effects of chemotherapy may contribute to the development of infections as well. Unlike CML, CLL does not transform into an acute blast cell leukemic form in its terminal phases.

12.1.4 TREATMENT

Management of CLL is based upon (1) recognition of the relatively indolent early course of the disease, (2) treatment of acute complications such as infection or autoimmune phenomena, when required, and (3) reservation of cytocidal chemotherapy for control of severe discomforting or disabling lymphadenopathy or splenomegaly, or progressive marrow infiltration with cytopenias. The number of circulating lymphocytes alone appears to be a poor indicator of need for chemotherapy.

Treatment of CLL is largely supportive. Infections are treated with appropriate antimicrobial agents. Autoimmune hemolytic anemia will generally respond to steroids (usually prednisone). When anemia, thrombocytopenia or organ discomfort is due to increased numbers of lymphocytes, chemotherapy is indicated. The chemotherapeutic agents most effective in CLL are the alkylating agents chlorambucil and cyclophosphamide.

12.2 Lymphomas

The lymphomas comprise a group of disorders characterized by abnormal proliferation of lymph node elements.

12.2.1 CLASSIFICATION AND PATHOGENESIS

The two major morphologically distinguishable cell types in lymphoid tissues are (1) lymphocytes and (2) histiocytes. Histiocytes are closely related to tissue macrophages and have features in common with monocytes and reticulum cells. Histiocytes are distinguished by their vesicular nuclei, nucleoli and abundant cytoplasm. The pathologic diagnosis of malignancy is based both on the morphology of the proliferative cells and on demonstration of destruction or obliteration of normal node architecture by lymphoma cells. The lymphomas are categorized by the histology of the malignant cell population, as revealed by lymph node biopsy (Table 12–1). *Poorly differentiated lymphocytic lymphomas* are composed of large immature lymphocytoid cells. In *well-differentiated lymphocytic lymphoma* the cells resemble normal small lymphocytes, although nodal architecture is disrupted. Nodal involvement in chronic lymphocytic leukemia is essentially indistinguishable from this pattern. The *histiocytic lymphomas* (reticulum cell sarcomas) also may be either well- or poorly differentiated in appearance, based on cell size, nuclear morphology and capacity for fiber formation and phagocytosis, two prominent histiocytic functions. *Mixed lymphocytic* and *histiocytic lymphomas* are not uncommon. All of the lymphomas may retain a *nodular* pattern or display *diffuse* infiltration of nodes.

A special form of lymphoma, *Hodgkin's disease,* is distinguished histologically by characteristic multinucleated giant cells (Reed-Sternberg cells), in addition to abnormal histiocytic and lymphocytic cells. Several histologic variants of Hodgkin's disease are defined by their content of histiocytic, lymphocytic and fibrous tissue elements (see Table 12–1). These are, according to current nomenclature:

1. *Lymphocytic predominance.* Abundant lymphocytes and/or histiocytes with sparse Reed-Sternberg cells.

2. *Nodular sclerosis.* Bands of collagenous connective tissue encircling nodular regions of lymphomatous tissue including Reed-Sternberg cells.

3. *Mixed cellularity type.* Marked pleocytosis including histiocytes, lymphocytes, granulocytes, plasma cells, fibroblasts and Reed-Sternberg cells.

4. *Lymphocytic depletion.* Diffuse fibrosis in association with increased numbers of histiocytes, a paucity of lymphocytes and the presence of Reed-Sternberg cells.

Several features have emerged as particularly useful in predicting the course and in designing a rational therapeutic program for the lymphomas. These are (1) anatomic extent of disease (staging), (2) histopathologic

TABLE 12–1.—CLASSIFICATION OF LYMPHOMAS

PREDOMINANT CELL TYPE	DISEASE*
Lymphocytic	Poorly differentiated lymphocytic lymphoma Well-differentiated lymphocytic lymphoma Hodgkin's disease, lymphocytic predominance Hodgkin's disease, nodular sclerosis
	Hodgkin's disease, mixed cellularity Lymphoma, mixed cellularity
Histiocytic	Histiocytic lymphoma Hodgkin's disease, lymphocytic depletion

*All of the non-Hodgkin lymphomas can be nodular or diffuse.

type and (3) systemic symptoms. These factors have been most explicitly defined in the case of the Hodgkin lymphomas; their implications for the non-Hodgkin types have yet to be fully evaluated.

12.2.2 ANATOMIC STAGING

The significance of accurately determining the anatomic extent of disease derives from studies on the natural history of Hodgkin's disease. In particular, it has become clear that this lymphoma spreads in a relatively predictable fashion along known patterns of lymphatic drainage from an apparently unicentric lymphatic origin. If the disease is limited to the lymphatic system and is relatively localized, radiotherapy with curative intent can be undertaken with excellent anticipation of success (see section 12.2.6). Disseminated, extralymphatic disease due presumably to vascular metastasis cannot be successfully treated with radiotherapy, and chemotherapy is indicated. Thus, optimal therapy depends on accurate initial staging. Incorrect staging can have disastrous consequences. The mistaken use of extensive radiotherapy, for example, for disease that has already spread beyond the lymphatic system can seriously compromise subsequent attempts to administer adequate chemotherapy because of the unavoidable and additive myelosuppressive effects of both x-irradiation and chemotherapy.

In the non-Hodgkin lymphomas, multiple foci and extranodal involvement are often present at the time of diagnosis and the pattern of spread of the disease is much less predictable. Dissemination to bone marrow and other nonlymphoid tissues is often evident early in the course of the disease when lymph node involvement is modest or even inapparent. It is hypothesized that in the non-Hodgkin lymphomas, either vascular spread of tumor occurs at an early time or the tumor is multicentric in origin.

Staging is of two types, clinical and pathologic. *Clinical staging* is based on the findings obtained by history, physical examination and noninvasive laboratory and radiologic evaluation. Four stages are presently recognized (Table 12–2). Stage I disease is defined as involvement of a single node or a contiguous group of nodes; Stage II disease involves two or more node-bearing areas above *or* below the diaphragm; in Stage III, nodes are involved both above *and* below the diaphragm. The spleen is defined as a lymph node region and is specifically designated (S). Stage IV disease is defined by the presence of extranodal involvement, e.g., bone, bone marrow and pulmonary and gastrointestinal infiltration. A *single* extralymphatic site, intimately associated with an involved lymph node, e.g., an isolated pelvic bone lesion adjacent to an involved inguinal node, is designated by a subscript E (meaning extranodal). The presence of a single extranodal site under these circumstances does not imply dissemination (Stage IV). The presence or absence of systemic (constitutional) symptoms is also determined as part of clinical staging; patients with fever, night sweats or weight loss of greater than 10% of body weight usually have more widespread disease and a poorer prognosis. The designation A following the stage number indicates that the patient is free of these systemic symptoms; B indicates that the patient has such symp-

TABLE 12–2.—STAGING OF LYMPHOMAS

STAGE	DEFINITION
I	Involvement of a single lymph node or lymph node region (e.g., the spleen).
II	Involvement of two or more node regions either above *or* below the diaphragm.
III	Involvement of lymph nodes or node regions both above *and* below the diaphragm.
IV	Involvement of one or more extralymphatic organs with or without lymph node involvement. The extralymphatic organs include liver, bone marrow, bone, pleura, lung, skin, central nervous system, etc. A *single* extralymphatic site contiguous with an involved lymph node is designated subscript E and does not indicate Stage IV disease if it is the only extralymphatic site.

toms. Pruritus is not a reliable indicator of the severity of disease and its presence or absence does not alter the classification. As an example of clinical staging, a patient with cervical and para-aortic lymph node involvement, splenomegaly and constitutional symptoms would be designated as having Stage IIIB (S) disease.

Clinical staging requires a detailed history to elicit systemic symptomatology (A or B disease) and a careful physical examination to determine the size and distribution of involved lymph node-bearing areas, and whether the liver and spleen are enlarged. Routine laboratory evaluation should include a complete blood count, platelet count, erythrocyte sedimentation rate, liver function tests, uric acid and blood urea nitrogen. A chest x-ray is required to detect enlarged hilar and mediastinal lymph nodes, or pleural or pulmonary parenchymal disease. An intravenous pyelogram can help screen for enlarged retroperitoneal nodes and may show ureteral deviation if significantly enlarged nodes are present. A negative pyelogram does not, however, exclude retroperitoneal nodal disease. A skeletal survey and radioactive bone scan are useful in determining if bone involvement exists; a bone marrow biopsy may detect dissemination to this site. Closed liver biopsy is often negative, even in the presence of liver involvement. Thus, a negative biopsy is not meaningful.

Bilateral lower extremity lymphangiography is useful for identifying tumor-bearing abdominal lymph nodes in the para-aortic and femoral lymph node regions. It is inadequate for defining nodes in the porta hepatis. In addition, there are significant numbers of both false positive and false negative lymphangiograms; thus, lymphangiograms usually are not used to stage the patient definitively. However, lymphangiograms are helpful in locating potentially involved nodes for biopsy at laparotomy. The dye persists in the nodes for a considerable period and may be useful in following the effect of treatment on lymph node size. Lymphangiograms are not done in patients with compromising pulmonary disease, since the dye, which enters the systemic circulation via the thoracic duct, can exacerbate previous pulmonary insufficiency when it enters the pulmonary vasculature.

Pathological staging depends upon the extent of disease, as defined by histologic examination of excised tissue. The diagnosis of lymphoma usually is first made by biopsy of an enlarged lymph node but also can be made from spleen or other involved organ samples. The diagnosis of lymphoma cannot be made without a properly evaluated biopsy regardless of the clinical presentation. Treatment decisions, particularly critical in Hodgkin's disease, depend on the extent of nodal and extranodal disease. An exploratory laparotomy including splenectomy, open liver biopsy and biopsy of nodes in the para-aortic, porta hepatis and other suspicious nodal areas is performed when the decision between curative radiotherapy and chemotherapy cannot otherwise be made. Splenectomy removes a potential site of disease and eliminates the need for radiation to the left upper quadrant, which inevitably includes potentially damaging radiation to the left kidney and left lower lobe of the lung. The size of the spleen is not a reliable indicator of the presence of splenic involvement; some enlarged spleens show no evidence of infiltration, whereas about 50% of normal-sized spleens demonstrate microscopic foci of disease. Pathologic examination of the spleen has another impact on prognosis, since liver disease is almost never seen without splenic involvement in Hodgkin's disease. The presence or absence of histologically proved splenic and abdominal node disease often determines the areas to which curative radiotherapy is given; total nodal irradiation (delivery of irradiation to central node-bearing areas both above and below the diaphragm; Fig. 12–1) may be given for extensive nodal disease, whereas only the supra-

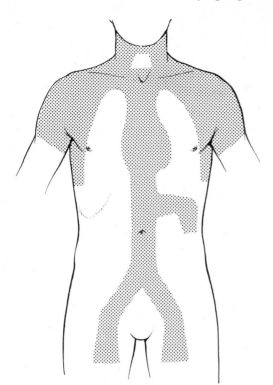

Fig. 12–1.—Anatomic extent of total nodal radiotherapy used in Hodgkin's disease. The stippled area indicates the sites irradiated.

or infradiaphragmatic fields may be irradiated for localized disease. Postsplenectomy infections appear to be a potential complication of this staging procedure in children, but not in adults. If Stage IV Hodgkin's disease is discovered during initial clinical evaluation (bone marrow, liver biopsy, bone scan), laparotomy is not indicated. At the present time it seems reasonable that pathologic staging by laparotomy with splenectomy be undertaken in most patients with Stage I, II or IIIA Hodgkin's disease in order to exclude Stage IV and to confirm the presence or absence of splenic and abdominal node disease.

The significance or usefulness of accurate staging in non-Hodgkin lymphomas has not been completely resolved. In these disorders less predictable progression of disease and the presence of disseminated disease at the time of diagnosis in the majority of patients make accurate staging much more difficult. In addition, radiotherapeutic cure of non-Hodgkin lymphomas is not nearly as common as in Hodgkin's disease, and chemotherapy also is less effective in these disorders.

12.2.3 HISTOPATHOLOGY

Histopathologic type often provides significant information related to extent of disease and prognosis in the lymphomas. In Hodgkin's disease, lymphocytic predominance and nodular sclerosis generally are more localized (Stages I and II), whereas lymphocytic depletion is often widespread and aggressive, with a correspondingly poorer prognosis for cure. The mixed cellularity class has an intermediate prognostic implication. Among the non-Hodgkin lymphomas, a nodular histology is associated with a better outlook than is diffuse disease in any of the cellular types. When lymphocytes predominate (lymphocytic lymphoma), the disease is often less aggressive and the chance for prolonged remission is relatively good. This is especially true when the malignant cell is a mature lymphocyte (well-differentiated lymphocytic lymphoma). When immature lymphocytes or lymphoblasts are the major cell types (poorly differentiated lymphocytic lymphoma), the prognosis is more guarded. In histiocytic lymphomas the disease is generally aggressive and the prognosis much less optimistic. Diffuse histiocytic lymphoma is more likely than all other lymphomas to present as extranodal disease, most commonly in the gastrointestinal tract or skin, less often in lung or bone.

12.2.4 OTHER CLINICAL AND LABORATORY FINDINGS

The usual presenting complaint in lymphoma of any type is lymphadenopathy, either localized or widespread. There may be fever (particularly common in Hodgkin's disease), pruritus, weight loss, anorexia or night sweats. Physical examination may reveal lymphadenopathy, hepatomegaly and/or splenomegaly. Clinical evaluation may fail in some cases to distinguish lymphoma from benign causes of lymphadenopathy. These include acute or chronic infections such as tuberculosis, toxoplasmosis, infectious mononucleosis and cat-scratch fever. In addition, sarcoidosis, collagen vascular diseases, autoimmune disorders, chronic lymphadenitis associated with diphenylhydantoin therapy and thyrotoxicosis may be associated with significant lymphadenopathy. It should be emphasized that the diagnosis of lymphoma can only be made by tissue biopsy reviewed by a competent pathologist.

In Hodgkin's disease there are often significant immunologic abnormalities involving delayed hypersensitivity reactions. Ig production usually is normal, but anergy (loss of normal skin hypersensitivity reactions, e.g., to purified protein derivative (PPD) or mumps antigens) is common. Anergy is more common in advanced disease and in the lymphocytic depletion type. Patients with Hodgkin's disease are more susceptible to opportunistic infections, including viruses (especially herpes zoster), fungi and protozoans.

12.2.5 THERAPY

In the lymphomas the goal of therapy should be clearly defined: Is it palliation or cure? In untreated patients at all stages of Hodgkin's disease, cure usually is attempted using intensive treatment with either radiotherapy or chemotherapy, or both. Upon relapse or progressive widespread disease, palliation may become the goal and less intensive treatment given. The initial treatment decision in Hodgkin's disease is critical, and ill-advised radiotherapy in disseminated disease may compromise the chances for successful chemotherapy. Patients who relapse after initial therapy with either chemotherapy or radiation may not be as responsive to

subsequent treatment and generally have a poorer prognosis than do untreated patients. These facts re-emphasize the importance of accurate staging prior to therapeutic decisions.

12.2.6 SPECIFIC THERAPY OF HODGKIN'S DISEASE

Stage I and II diseases are treated with radiotherapy either to all central lymph node-bearing areas (total nodal radiotherapy) or to the so-called extended field, which excludes lymph node areas remote from the primary site of involvement (i.e., exclusion of pelvic nodes in a patient with IA disease localized to the supraclavicular region). An overall 5-year disease-free remission rate of over 90% can be expected in Stage I disease and close to this in Stage IIA disease treated with adequate radiotherapy. The management of patients with IIB and III disease is still controversial. Total nodal radiotherapy alone results in complete remissions in approximately 40–70% of patients 3 years after diagnosis and treatment. However, programs using combination chemotherapy also approach this degree of effectiveness. Therefore, in Stage III disease controlled clinical trials are in progress comparing radiotherapy and multiple drug chemotherapy, either alone or in combination, to determine optimal management. Stage IV disease is treated primarily with chemotherapy since extranodal disease cannot be safely and effectively treated by radiotherapy. In Stage III or IV Hodgkin's disease, combination chemotherapy alone is very effective in inducing remissions of long duration. The combination of prednisone, vincristine, procarbazine and nitrogen mustard (MOPP) has been the best studied and is greatly superior to sequential use of single agents. Courses of MOPP given over a 6-month period have produced an 80% remission rate and an average 42-month disease-free remission in previously untreated patients with Stage IIIB or IV disease. Remissions in previously treated patients are generally of shorter duration but can be expected in 50–60% of cases. Vinblastine, bleomycin, adriamycin and the nitrosoureas are additional useful agents in treatment of disease refractory to MOPP. The role of long-term maintenance therapy has not yet been clearly defined.

12.2.7 SPECIFIC THERAPY OF NON-HODGKIN LYMPHOMAS

Diffuse histiocytic lymphoma is generally resistant to therapy. Most patients succumb within 1 year of diagnosis. In a minority of patients with localized disease, radiotherapy may result in extended remission or cure. In Stage III and IV diseases, treatment usually includes combinations of radiotherapy and chemotherapy. The most effective agents in use today are vincristine, cyclophosphamide, bleomycin, adriamycin and the steroids.

Well-differentiated diffuse lymphocytic lymphosarcoma usually has disseminated by the time of diagnosis. Attempts at cure by radiotherapy are confined to early stages. Stage III and IV diseases are treated with chemotherapy, usually given when the patient becomes symptomatic or the disease shows progression. Vincristine, cyclophosphamide and prednisone are used in combination to induce remission. Asymptomatic, nonprogressive disease, even though widespread, may remain stable, without treatment, for years. Poorly differentiated lymphocytic lymphosarcoma is more aggressive, has a poorer prognosis and is usually treated with chemotherapy.

Nodular lymphomas (giant follicular lymphomas) generally are slowly progressive disorders. Nodular lymphocytic lymphoma has a better prognosis than does nodular histiocytic disease. Radiotherapy is the treatment of choice for these radiosensitive tumors when they are localized. Chemotherapy may be useful in controlling more disseminated disease associated with systemic symptomatology.

12.3 Histiocytic Infiltrations Related to Lymphomas

Histiocytic medullary reticulosis is associated with histiocyte infiltration in many organs. Characteristically there are lymphadenopathy and hepatosplenomegaly. Lymph node biopsy reveals proliferation of histiocytes, which are frequently engaged in erythrophagocytosis. Anemia, thrombocytopenia and leukopenia are common. The disorder is resistant to the chemotherapeutic agents currently used.

The *Sézary syndrome* describes the association of certain dermatologic conditions, commonly exfoliative dermatitis and erythroderma, with the finding of abnormal lymphocytoid (Sézary) cells in the circulating blood. Sézary cells characteristically have deeply convoluted nuclei with many clefts and may be present in large numbers in the peripheral blood. Peripheral lymphadenopathy may be present and may be either infiltrative or due to chronic lymphadenitis accompanying the dermatologic abnormalities. The relationship of this disorder to *mycosis fungoides,* a lymphoma-like disease of the skin, is unclear. In this latter disorder the skin is infiltrated by a mixed cell population including lymphoreticular cells, eosinophils, granulocytes and plasma cells. Mycosis fungoides is often found in association with systemic lymphoma.

13

Plasma Cell Dyscrasias and Immunoglobulin Diseases

13.1 Origin and Function of Plasma Cells

PLASMA CELLS are believed to derive from lymphocytes, presumably of the B type (see section 9.3.2). Plasma cell proliferation normally occurs in lymph nodes, spleen and bone marrow under the stimulus of antigenic substances. Less commonly, during intense antigenic stimulation, plasma cells may appear transiently in the blood. Each clone of lymphocytes and plasma cells produces one or, at most, a small number of Ig.

13.2 Immunoglobulins

Ig molecules are of several types. Each type contains four polypeptide chains. Two of the polypeptide chains are heavy (H) chains and have 450 amino acids and a molecular weight of 52,000. Two other chains, light (L) chains, contain approximately 215 amino acids and have a molecular weight of 22,000. The basic molecular structure and function of IgG and IgM have been discussed in a previous section (6.4). IgA, IgD and IgE are each distinguished by unique heavy chains (α, δ and ϵ, respectively) and characteristic biologic properties. IgA is found in external secretions; IgE is implicated in allergic reactions; the function of IgD remains obscure.

By cellulose acetate electrophoresis at pH 8, all Ig migrate with the mobility of β or γ globulins (Fig. 13–1); all except IgM have sedimentation coefficients between omission 6.5 and 8S, whereas IgM is considerably larger (18S). Antisera prepared against each

110

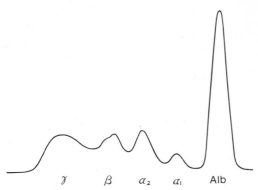

Fig. 13–1.—Normal serum protein electrophoretic pattern. $\gamma = \gamma$ globulins; $\beta = \beta$ globulins; $\alpha = \alpha$ globulins; Alb = albumin. This is a densitometry tracing of the pattern obtained by electrophoresis of serum on cellulose acetate.

of the specific Ig subclasses are used to detect and quantitate each type of Ig.

Disorders of Ig production may be associated with diffuse hyper- or hypogammaglobulinemia or with overproduction of a unique molecular species of Ig, producing a

Fig. 13–2.—Serum protein electrophoretic pattern in a patient with multiple myeloma. $\gamma = \gamma$ globulins; $\beta = \beta$ globulins; $\alpha = \alpha$ globulins; Alb = albumin. This is a densitometry tracing of electrophoresis of serum using cellulose acetate. The increase in size and sharp contour of the γ peak indicates the presence of a "γ spike" characteristic of multiple myeloma.

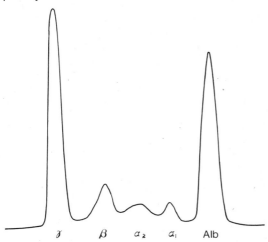

homogeneous "spike" of Ig on plasma protein electrophoresis (Fig. 13–2). Normal populations of plasma cells and plasma cells associated with reactive immune responses produce Ig molecules with both κ and λ chains; a clone of malignant plasma cells produces Ig displaying either κ or λ chains, but not both. When hypergammaglobulinemia is associated with a discrete class of Ig with a single type of L chain (either κ or λ), the Ig is said to be *monoclonal* (produced by the progeny of a single cell). The sharp peak of Ig recognized on electrophoresis and characterized by immunodiffusion is called a monoclonal spike. Monoclonal gammopathies may be of any Ig class but most commonly involve IgG or IgM.

13.3 Plasma Cell Dyscrasias

The plasma cell dyscrasias are a group of disorders in which a clone of Ig-producing cells generates a monoclonal gammopathy. Variants of this group of disorders are described in which (1) the proliferation of plasma cells is invasive, (2) a monoclonal Ig is the only evidence of disease and (3) only H or L chains or even no Ig components at all are produced by the abnormal clone of cells.

In most cases the abnormal plasma cell clone produces equal amounts of H and L chains. However, in some cases there is a relative excess production of either H or L chains. Most often, when unbalanced synthesis occurs, it is the L chains that are present in excess. When L chains, also called Bence-Jones protein, are produced in excess of H chains, they circulate in the peripheral blood and can be demonstrated by immunoprecipitation using antibodies specifically directed against either κ or λ L chains. Bence-Jones protein, in contrast to complete Ig molecules, traverse the glomerulus and are concentrated in the urine. The presence of Bence-Jones protein in the urine can be identified by its unique property of precipitating upon heating to 50–60 C and of reversion into solution at 90–95 C. Bence-Jones protein most often can be demonstrated by electrophoresis of urinary protein even when small amounts are present. Commonly used tests for urine protein (i.e., Albumistix) will not reliably detect Bence-Jones protein; heat or acid precipitation tests must be used. When the abnormal plasma cells produce both L and H chains, but produce L chains in excess, an abnormal Ig spike will be seen in the serum, and Bence-Jones protein will be found in urine.

Plasma cell dyscrasia associated with destructive bone lesions is called *multiple myeloma* or *plasma cell myeloma*. This disorder is characterized by (1) an increase in malignant plasma cells in bone marrow and, in some instances, in other organs; (2) destructive bone lesions due to the expansive and invasive properties of these plasma cells and (3) the presence of a monoclonal Ig, containing either κ or λ L chains.

13.3.1 CLINICAL AND HEMATOLOGIC FINDINGS

The initial complaint of the majority of patients with multiple myeloma is bone pain. Symptoms of anemia also may be present. Physical examination may demonstrate areas of bone tenderness. Anemia becomes increasingly common as the disease progresses; it is normocytic and normochromic and is due to decreased production in the marrow. Rouleaux formation due to elevated Ig levels may be prominent and accounts for the extremely rapid sedimentation rate observed in many instances. The WBC count is most often normal, although it may also be low, as may be the platelet count. Plasma cells are rarely seen on peripheral blood examination. Radiologic findings characteristically include multiple osteolytic lesions of the skeleton, although solitary lesions can occur. Frequently involved areas include the rib cage, sternum, spine and skull; occasionally the bone lesions are indistinguishable from benign osteoporosis. The radiographic findings also may resemble other tumors involving bone. Examination of bone marrow often shows an increase in plasma cells and may reveal sheets of these cells. Sheets of plasma cells strongly suggest the diagnosis of multiple myeloma. Although the malignant cells appear immature and display abnormal nuclear morphology, the cytology of plasma cells is not diagnostic of malignancy.

13.3.2 DIAGNOSIS

The diagnosis of multiple myeloma is established when bone lesions are found in association with a serum or urine monoclonal Ig or Bence-Jones protein. In about 25% of cases, only Bence-Jones proteinuria is found; approximately half of these cases show κ-type Bence-Jones protein and the rest show λ chains. Approximately 50% of cases of myeloma are associated with monoclonal IgG spikes and, in approximately half of these, Bence-Jones proteinuria is present as well. Another 20% of patients with myeloma have IgA spikes, and approximately one third of these patients also have Bence-Jones proteinuria.

13.3.3 DIFFERENTIAL DIAGNOSIS

Plasmacytosis in the bone marrow may occur in a variety of benign conditions including chronic infection, hepatitis and cirrhosis. Bone lesions similar to those found in multiple myeloma also may occur in metastatic carcinoma, severe osteoporosis and hyperparathyroidism. It may be necessary to biopsy the bone lesion to determine the nature of the underlying disorder. Multiple myeloma also must be distinguished from benign monoclonal gammopathies unassociated with bone lesions, from macroglobulinemia and from H chain disease (see below).

13.3.4 SPECIAL PROBLEMS IN MULTIPLE MYELOMA

1. *Diffuse hypogammoglobulinemia.* Despite the increased total Ig due to the abnormal monoclonal protein, normal Ig and antibody levels in myeloma usually are depressed. An increased incidence of bacterial

infections is common. Pneumococcal infections are most common, but gram-negative infection also is recognized.

2. *Hypercalcemia.* Hypercalcemia is a frequent complication of myeloma and must be strongly suspected, especially in patients confined to bed because of bone pain. Prompt treatment of hypercalcemia is essential to forestall renal lithiasis, nephrocalcinosis and renal failure as well as neurologic sequelae of hypercalcemia.

3. *Renal failure.* Renal failure occurs in many patients with multiple myeloma either early in the course of disease or during its progression. A characteristic renal lesion in multiple myeloma is tubular degeneration associated with proteinuria and azotemia. The relationship between Bence-Jones proteinuria and the development of renal failure is unclear. Bence-Jones protein has been identified in the cytoplasm of tubular cells.

4. *Hyperviscosity.* In certain plasma cell myelomas, abnormal Ig may form large molecular weight aggregates and markedly increase the blood viscosity. The symptoms of hyperviscosity include neurologic deficits and circulatory dysfunction. Hyperviscosity syndromes are more commonly associated with monoclonal IgM and macroglobulinemia (see section 13.5).

5. *Acute neurologic deficits.* Cord compression, due to plasmacytoma or to vertebral collapse, may necessitate emergency laminectomy in order to avoid paraplegia. Patients with collapsed vertebrae must be watched closely for development of this complication.

6. *Amyloidosis.* This usually is a late complication in the course of multiple myeloma and involves the deposition of eosinophilic material in many organs. Some amyloid deposits represent complexes of Ig L chains and tissue components. The pattern of organ involvement in myeloma-associated amyloidosis may be either (1) of the "primary" type in which the gastrointestinal tract, cardiac muscle and peripheral nerves are affected (the latter associated with the carpal tunnel syndrome); or (2) of the "sec-

ondary" type involving the kidneys, liver and spleen. Rectal and gum biopsy may be useful in leading to a diagnosis of primary amyloidosis.

7. *Cryoglobulins.* These may be associated with plasma cell dyscrasias. Cryoglobulins are Ig molecules that precipitate in the cold. Cryoglobulinemia may be accompanied by Raynaud's phenomenon and, in more severe cases, by gangrene.

8. *Relation to other neoplasms.* On rare occasions plasma cell leukemia may intervene in the course of a plasma cell dyscrasia. The symptoms and signs are similar to those present in other acute leukemias and may include systemic symptoms, hepatosplenomegaly, anemia and thrombocytopenia. The peripheral blood contains immature plasma cells. Bence-Jones protein and abnormal serum Ig may occur, as in myeloma. It is also reported that the incidence of second independent tumors is higher in patients with multiple myeloma than it is in the general population. Carcinomas of the colon, breast and biliary tract occur most frequently. Acute leukemia also has been reported as the terminal phase in some patients with myeloma. A relationship between these neoplasms and the alkylating agents used to treat the myeloma has been suggested but is unproved to date.

13.3.5 TREATMENT

Treatment is of two types: (1) supportive, and (2) using specific chemotherapy and x-irradiation. Patients with extensive bone lesions tend to develop hypercalcemia at bed rest and this complication should be treated prophylactically by adequate mobilization and hydration. When hypercalcemia occurs despite these measures, saline diuresis and steroid therapy are most useful. In addition, oral phosphate, phosphate infusions and mithramycin are effective agents for lowering calcium levels.

Plasma cell tumors are generally sensitive to radiotherapy. Localized plasmacytomas, in bone or elsewhere, can be treated by radiotherapy. When the lesions are extensive and none is uniquely severe or life threatening, a course of chemotherapy should be initiated as early as possible. The total body tumor cell load in myeloma usually is very large, and complete eradication is difficult. However, significant, rapid relief of symptoms can accompany adequate doses of effective chemotherapy. The most effective agents are phenylalanine mustard (PAM) and cyclophosphamide, both alkylating agents. It is usually necessary to achieve mild leukopenia in order to be certain that an adequate amount of drug is being given. The major side-effect of both drugs is pancytopenia due to bone marrow suppression. In addition, cyclophosphamide can cause severe hemorrhagic cystitis. Both cyclophosphamide and PAM will produce remission in approximately 50–60% of patients with multiple myeloma. However, only about half of patients so treated are still alive after 3 years. The major clinical and laboratory responses seen with these agents are relief of bone pain, decrease in level of abnormal Ig in serum and of Bence-Jones protein (if present), increase in hemoglobin concentration and subsidence of hypercalcemia. Healing of bone lesions on x-ray usually is not seen even in responding patients. Adrenal steroids appear to act synergistically with cyclophosphamide or PAM. The nitrosoureas also show promise in therapy of multiple myeloma.

13.4 Plasma Cell Dyscrasias without Bone Lesions (Benign Monoclonal Gammopathy)

A monoclonal Ig, the product of a unique population of plasma cells, does not necessarily indicate the presence of multiple myeloma. Benign monoclonal gammopathies are associated with a variety of conditions and may be either transient or persistent. Some are of little or no clinical significance, whereas others are serious illnesses in which monoclonal gammopathy is an incidental finding.

Transient benign monoclonal hyperglob-ulinemia has been reported as a reaction to drugs, especially the sulfonamides. The amount of abnormal protein usually does not exceed 1 gm % and spontaneously regresses.

Persistent benign monoclonal hyperglobulinemia has been reported with chronic inflammatory and infectious processes including tuberculosis, chronic biliary tract disease, nephritis and rheumatoid arthritis, as well as in association with carcinomas of the colon, breast and biliary tract and in patients with Gaucher's disease, familial hypercholesterolemia and xanthomatosis. It has been suggested that in these disorders, chronic stimulation of Ig-producing cells by chronic inflammatory disease or by tumor stimulates the emergence of a clone of plasma cells. Waldenström has shown that up to 3% of patients over 70 years old have monoclonal Ig spikes of unknown significance and unassociated with bone lesions.

13.5 Waldenström's Macroglobulinemia

Waldenström's macroglobulinemia is associated with a monoclonal increase in IgM (macroglobulin) due presumably to monoclonal lymphoid cell proliferation. Lymphadenopathy and hepatosplenomegaly are common, whereas osteolytic lesions are rare. Symptoms usually are related to hyperviscosity any may include a variety of neurologic manifestations, with paralysis, sensory symptoms or disordered consciousness. Vascular lesions with both thrombosis and hemorrhage and, in more severe cases, with gangrene of extremities also occur. Coagulation disorders due to interaction of IgM proteins with specific coagulation factors, especially factors I (fibrinogen), II (prothrombin), V and VII are reported (see section 18.2.6). Bence-Jones proteinuria has been described and may be associated with azotemia. The peripheral blood usually reveals a normochromic normocytic anemia, rouleaux formation and a relative lymphocytosis. The lymphocytes may display morphologic features resembling plasma cells. The bone marrow usually demonstrates the presence of similar abnormal lymphocytes.

The diagnosis requires the combination of monoclonal IgM in the serum in association with lymphoid cell proliferation. Primary macroglobulinemia must be distinquished from lymphoproliferative disorders, such as chronic lymphocytic leukemia or lymphosarcoma cell leukemia, and from secondary macroglobulinemia associated with a variety of tumors.

Use of chlorambucil, an alkylating agent, is the treatment of choice in this disorder and often produces sustained remission. The drug should be continued indefinitely since cessation of therapy is regularly associated with relapse. Patients may become refractory to chemotherapy and develop progressive anemia, complications of hyperviscosity, hemorrhage or infection.

13.6 Heavy Chain Diseases

In these disorders, there is monoclonal production of the H chains or H chain fragments.

IgG H chain disease is associated with fever, susceptibility to bacterial infection, lymphadenopathy and hepatosplenomegaly. Laboratory examination reveals anemia, leukopenia and thrombocytopenia. Bone marrow aspiration shows increased plasma cells and lymphocytes. Immunoelectrophoretic studies indicate that the abnormal protein is a homogeneous IgG H chain fragment. The treatment of H chain disease with cyclophosphamide, PAM and steroids has been disappointing. Death occurs usually from uncontrollable infection.

In *IgA H chain disease* there is an abnormal monoclonal α chain (the H chain of IgA). The disease usually presents with evidence of an abdominal lymphoma. Symptoms include chronic diarrhea, malabsorption and lymphomatous infiltration in the small intes-

tine and mesenteric regions. The presence of IgA H chains in serum provides the diagnosis. In contrast to IgG H chain disease, IgA H chains usually are not found in urine, presumably because they aggregate and cannot pass the renal glomerulus. Most patients described to date have been Sephardic Jews or Israeli Arabs.

The single patient reported with *IgM H chain disease* had the clinical picture of chronic lymphocytic leukemia. The patient subsequently developed amyloidosis and the carpal tunnel syndrome. The abnormal protein was found only in serum, not in urine.

13.7 Ig Deficiency Diseases

A variety of inherited disorders of Ig production have been described. These include the *Di George syndrome;* a sex-linked congenital agammaglobulinemia *(Bruton type);* a sex-linked lymphopenic agammaglobulinemia and *Swiss-type* lymphopenic agammaglobulinemia. Agammaglobulinemia also is associated with thymoma. The *Wiscott-Aldrich syndrome* is associated with IgM deficiency, eczema and thrombocytopenia. *Ataxia-telangiectasia* combines decreased IgA production with ataxia, telangiectases and an increased incidence of lymphoreticular neoplasms. Hypogammaglobulinemia also can be acquired and is regularly observed in chronic lymphocytic leukemia, other lymphoid neoplasms and plasma cell dyscrasias.

Patients with any of the hypogammaglobulinemias may experience recurrent episodes of infections often caused by indigenous organisms (i.e., common bacteria of the nasopharynx or gastrointestinal tract), including pneumococci, *Haemophilus influenzae* and streptococci, as well as by fungal and viral agents. Pooled gamma globulin may be given to patients with hypogammaglobulinemia to prevent recurrent infections.

14

Hemostasis: Normal Mechanisms

14.1 Introduction

THE SUCCESSFUL MANAGEMENT of patients with hemorrhagic disorders depends on accurate diagnosis. Correct diagnosis and rational therapy depend on an understanding of the normal mechanisms for preserving hemostasis. Knowledge of the normal physiology is incomplete but nevertheless sufficiently developed to permit understanding of the diagnostic tests and available therapeutic measures.

Blood loss can occur only when the vessel wall is interrupted or rendered permeable to red cells. The rate of bleeding depends on the size and number of injured vessels and on the pressure in them. From a physical point of view, bleeding stops (1) if the pressure inside and outside of the damaged vessel is equalized, or (2) if the hole in the vessel is occluded by solid or very viscous material.

Pressure equalization can be produced by a rise in external pressure (e.g., hematoma) or by a fall in pressure inside the vessel, which may be local, or general (as in shock). Occlusion of the hole may be achieved by a ligature, by a mass of fibrin, aggregated platelets and cells or by active constriction of the vessel at the site of injury. The relative importance of these factors varies greatly according to the type of injury and the size of the vessels involved. Constriction may persist as a powerful spasm in large vessels for 20 minutes or more; in smaller vessels it usually passes off in 5–10 minutes and in capillaries it is of little or no importance. Constriction is produced by direct injury, by chemical or nervous stimulation or by the presence of shed blood or agglutinated platelets. The precise biochemical stimuli responsible for vasoconstriction have not been securely identified.

14.2 Normal Hemostatic Mechanisms

Normal hemostasis comprises mechanisms operative immediately following the injury and those acting over a longer period to maintain hemostasis.

The *immediate* mechanism consists principally of two components: (1) vasoconstriction due to active contraction of the muscle of the vessel wall, and (2) plug formation by masses of agglutinated platelets.

The *maintenance* mechanism consists of the fibrin clot, the product of the reactions of the coagulation system.

Platelet plug formation is especially important in capillary hemostasis, whereas vasoconstriction and the fibrin clot seem to be more important in large vessel hemostasis. The several mechanisms involved in achieving normal hemostasis are interconnected at several points, but for the sake of clarity each will be described as a separate entity.

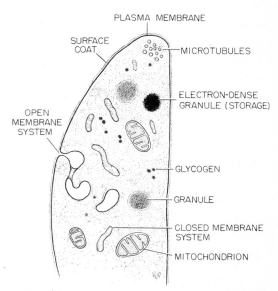

Fig. 14–1.—Platelet morphology. Schematic drawing of an electron micrograph of a section through a platelet.

14.3 Platelets

14.3.1 STRUCTURE

By light microscopy normal platelets are anucleate bodies about $2-3$ μ in diameter; they stain light blue and contain a varying number of small purple-red granules. With the electron microscope a distinct plasma membrane is clearly seen (Fig. 14–1). Outside of the plasma membrane is a surface coat of acid mucopolysaccharide.

The platelet plasma membrane is unique in that it possesses receptors that react with thrombin. The submembranous area and cytoplasm contain the contractile protein actomyosin (also termed thrombosthenin) in the form of a number of fibrous elements. In the submembranous area, microtubules form a cytoskeleton, which maintains the flattened disk shape of the platelet. Microfilaments in the cytoplasm are responsible for granule movement and fusion during aggregation.

Platelets contain vacuoles, vesicles and electron-dense granules, the chemical nature and functions of which are still poorly understood. Some of these structures must be lysosomes, since platelets contain lysosomal enzymes, e.g., acid phosphatase, cathepsin and glucuronidase, whereas others may be phagocytic vacuoles. Serotonin has been identified in the electron-dense granules. Serotonin is not synthesized in platelet precursors (megakaryocytes) but rather in argentaffin cells in the gastrointestinal mucosa. Released presumably in trace amounts into the plasma, it is concentrated within the platelet by an active process requiring energy. Still other vacuoles represent infoldings of the surface membrane cut in cross-section, the so-called surface-connecting system.

The platelets also contain mitochondria, glycogen and occasionally inclusions of lipid. Ribosomes have been detected, consistent with evidence that the platelet has a limited protein synthetic capacity. Platelets have an active intermediary metabolism; they generate ATP from both glycolysis and the tricarboxylic acid cycle and can synthesize glycogen and lipid.

14.3.2 DISTRIBUTION AND FATE OF PLATELETS

Platelets are formed in the marrow and released into the circulation. At any moment, about 80% of platelets are circulating and 20% are in the spleen. Platelets move freely between these two pools. If the spleen enlarges markedly, the distribution shifts: up to 80% of platelets may be pooled in a large spleen. Survival curves of platelets labeled with ^{51}Cr are linear and indicate that platelets become senescent and die after a finite life span of about 10 days (Fig. 14–2). However, survival curves of platelets with radiolabeled diisopropylfluorophosphate are curvilinear and indicate random destruction of platelets at a rate giving an intravascular $t^{1/2}$ of $3 – 4^{1/2}$ days. Which pattern most closely reflects physiologic platelet turnover is not yet clear. In a normal individual some platelets probably die of senescence after $7 – 14$ days, whereas other platelets (possibly a greater proportion of younger platelets) are consumed in repairing the minor vascular injuries of daily life. There is some evidence

Fig. 14–2.—Survival in the circulation of platelets labeled with ^{51}Cr in a normal individual and in a patient with idiopathic thrombocytopenic purpura (ITP).

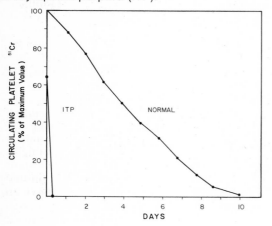

that younger platelets are larger, are physiologically more active and have higher enzyme concentrations than do old platelets. However, his distinction is most apparent when thrombopoiesis is accelerated in response to increased platelet destruction.

In the thrombocytopenia due to increased platelet destruction, the destruction is random. Senescent platelets are probably removed by the reticuloendothelial system. Damaged platelets may be removed primarily in the spleen or in both spleen and liver. The bone marrow does not contain a reserve of platelets. If circulating platelets are rapidly destroyed or lost, thrombocytopenia will persist for several days until enough new platelets are formed to correct it.

One or more humoral factors govern normal platelet production. A patient has been described with a chronic severe thrombocytopenia that could be temporarily corrected by transfusion of normal plasma. This patient apparently lacked a plasma factor, thrombopoietin, necessary for normal platelet production. Our understanding of the humoral control of platelet production remains, however, in its infancy.

14.3.3 PLATELET FUNCTION IN HEMOSTASIS

The contribution of the platelet to hemostasis is in the formation of the platelet plug and in promotion of thrombin production. Platelet plug formation may be divided into a number of stages (Fig. 14–3).

1. *Adhesion.* Platelets adhere to subendothelial structures exposed by trauma. Such structures include collagen fibers and basement membrane (Fig. 14–4). The presence of regularly spaced free amino groups on the collagen molecule is critical for platelet adhesion. In addition, a number of plasma proteins, including fibrinogen and "von Willebrand" factor, are required for normal platelet adhesion.

2. *Aggregation.* Adenosine diphosphate (ADP) released from the storage granules of

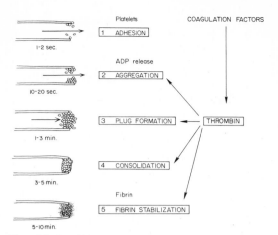

Fig. 14-3.—Formation of a hemostatic plug. Stages in the formation of a hemostatic plug are shown following transection of a small vessel. ADP = adenosine diphosphate.

adherent platelets causes additional platelets to aggregate at the site of a vascular injury. The mechanism of ADP action is as yet unsolved. ADP is discharged from platelet storage granules by an active process possibly stimulated by the combined action of collagen and thrombin.

ADP release and platelet aggregation induced by thrombin are inhibited by substances that increase the cyclic adenosine-3',5'-monophosphate (cyclic AMP) level of the platelet. These agents include a prostaglandin, which increases the activity of adenyl cyclase; an enzyme, which converts ATP to cyclic AMP; and theophylline, which inhibits phosphodiesterase, the enzyme that breaks down cyclic AMP. Epinephrine, on the other hand, which facilitates platelet aggregation, lowers platelet cyclic AMP levels. Recent studies indicate that intermediates of prostaglandin synthesis play a major role in mediating the release reaction and second-phase aggregation. When platelets are stimulated by a release-inducer, the enzyme *cyclo-oxygenase* converts arachidonic acid to a labile endoperoxide intermediate in prostaglandin synthesis. This endoperoxide, termed *Thromboxane A$_2$,* directly induces the release reaction.

The formation of platelet plugs is responsible for the rapid cessation of bleeding from ruptured capillaries and small vessels. The integrity of the platelet plug-forming mechanism is tested by measuring the bleeding time. A commonly used test for measuring bleeding time, termed the Ivy bleeding time, is performed by measuring the time taken for bleeding to cease from three 1 mm × 1 cm incisions in an avascular area of the forearm. Venous return is obstructed by a blood pressure cuff over the upper forearm, set at 40 mm Hg pressure. The bleeding time is normal in disorders of the coagulation system but is abnormal in the presence of severe thrombocytopenia, defects of platelet function, deficiency of the von Willebrand plasma protein or total absence of blood fibrinogen. Generally, clinically significant platelet function defects are found only if the bleeding time is prolonged. The normal platelet count is 150,000–400,000 cu mm, and the most accurate method of counting platelets is by

Fig. 14-4.—Schematic drawing of a section through the wall of a large vessel. E = endothelial cell; BM = basement membrane; Mf = microfibrils; CF = collagen fiber.

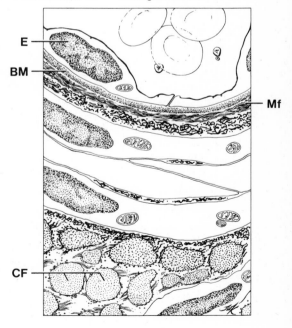

TABLE 14–1.—PATHOPHYSIOLOGY OF HEMOSTATIC DEFECTS

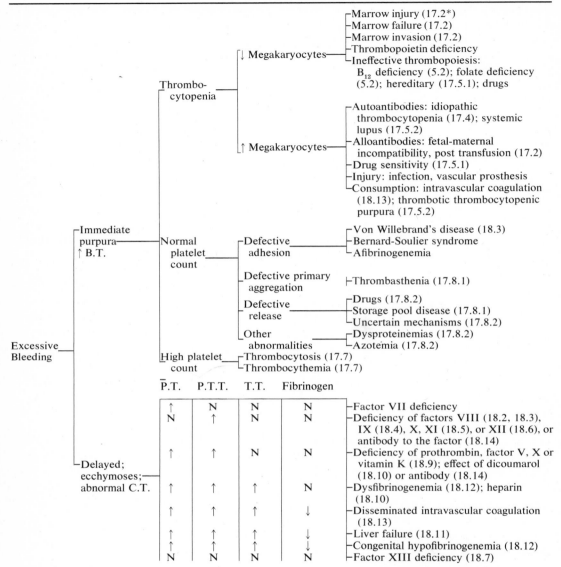

Excessive Bleeding

- Immediate purpura; ↑ B.T.
  - Thrombocytopenia
    - ↓ Megakaryocytes
      - Marrow injury (17.2*)
      - Marrow failure (17.2)
      - Marrow invasion (17.2)
      - Thrombopoietin deficiency
      - Ineffective thrombopoiesis: B_{12} deficiency (5.2); folate deficiency (5.2); hereditary (17.5.1); drugs
    - ↑ Megakaryocytes
      - Autoantibodies: idiopathic thrombocytopenia (17.4); systemic lupus (17.5.2)
      - Alloantibodies: fetal-maternal incompatibility, post transfusion (17.2)
      - Drug sensitivity (17.5.1)
      - Injury: infection, vascular prosthesis
      - Consumption: intravascular coagulation (18.13); thrombotic thrombocytopenic purpura (17.5.2)
  - Normal platelet count
    - Defective adhesion
      - Von Willebrand's disease (18.3)
      - Bernard-Soulier syndrome
      - Afibrinogenemia
    - Defective primary aggregation
      - Thrombasthenia (17.8.1)
    - Defective release
      - Drugs (17.8.2)
      - Storage pool disease (17.8.1)
      - Uncertain mechanisms (17.8.2)
    - Other abnormalities
      - Dysproteinemias (17.8.2)
      - Azotemia (17.8.2)
  - High platelet count
    - Thrombocytosis (17.7)
    - Thrombocythemia (17.7)
- Delayed; ecchymoses; abnormal C.T.

P.T.	P.T.T.	T.T.	Fibrinogen	
↑	N	N	N	Factor VII deficiency
N	↑	N	N	Deficiency of factors VIII (18.2, 18.3), IX (18.4), X, XI (18.5), or XII (18.6), or antibody to the factor (18.14)
↑	↑	N	N	Deficiency of prothrombin, factor V, X or vitamin K (18.9); effect of dicoumarol (18.10) or antibody (18.14)
↑	↑	↑	N	Dysfibrinogenemia (18.12); heparin (18.10)
↑	↑	↑	↓	Disseminated intravascular coagulation (18.13)
↑	↑	↑	↓	Liver failure (18.11)
↑	↑	↑	↓	Congenital hypofibrinogenemia (18.12)
N	N	N	N	Factor XIII deficiency (18.7)

*The numbers in parentheses refer to sections of the text in which a discussion relevant to each mechanism may be found. Where no reference is provided, the discussion lies outside the scope of this introductory text.

Abbreviations: N, normal; ↓ decreased; ↑ increased or prolonged; B.T., bleeding time; C.T., clotting tests; P.T., prothrombin time; P.T.T., partial thromboplastin; T.T., thrombin time.

phase-contrast microscopy. An estimate of platelet number may be made by examination of the stained peripheral blood smear. In the presence of a normal red cell count, 1 platelet/20 RBC is equivalent to a platelet count of 250,000/cu mm. Platelet aggregation may be studied by recording the increase in light transmitted through a cuvet containing continuously stirred platelet-rich plasma when aggregating agents are added to the plasma. The aggregating agents usually tested are collagen, norepinephrine, ADP, thrombin and the antibiotic, ristocetin.

3. *Platelet fusion (plug formation)*. This results from the action of thrombin produced by the coagulation mechanism. Fibrin, also a product of thrombin action, and fused platelets form a stable hemostatic plug. Platelets themselves participate in clotting reactions that lead to thrombin formation by providing "platelet factor 3" activity. This coagulation factor is actually the platelet membrane itself in a suitable configuration on which the coagulation enzymes and substrates can interact and promote clot formation. The platelet membrane surface promotes the coagulation reactions only after the platelets have aggregated. Hence, a defect in platelet aggregation will be detected as a defect in platelet factor 3 activity.

4. *Clot retraction (consolidation)*. This is the final stage of hemostatic plug formation. Platelets, probably by the action of thrombosthenin, pull the fibrin threads of the clot into a contracted volume and express the fluid trapped in the clot. Clot retraction is readily tested by adding thrombin to platelet-rich plasma and noting the extent of clot retraction 1 hour later. The retraction of clots in whole blood can similarly be evaluated. Clot retraction is defective in a severe congenital defect of platelet function, termed thrombasthenia. The reason for defective retraction in this disorder is not known; platelet thrombosthenin is normal. Clot retraction is also defective when either the platelet count or the concentration of fibrinogen is very low.

5. *Fibrin stabilization*. Fibrin, produced by thrombin action on fibrinogen, is cross-linked by covalent peptide bonds and contributes to the formation of a stable hemostatic plug.

14.4 Blood Coagulation

The two main functions of the blood coagulation mechanism are (1) production of thrombin, which stabilizes the platelet plug, and (2) formation of the fibrin clot, which mechanically blocks the flow of blood through ruptured vessels. A hemorrhagic diathesis may result from deficient activity of one or more coagulation factors or from inhibition of coagulation. Coagulation factor deficiencies may result from decreased production or from production of an abnormal protein with defective biologic activity or excessively rapid catabolism. Impaired production of coagulation factor activities may have a genetic basis or may be due to acquired disease, such as vitamin K deficiency or severe liver disease. Increased catabolism of coagulation factors may result from an increased rate of intravascular proteolysis.

Inhibition of coagulation may result from reduced concentration of a specific factor due to antibody to the precursor factor or due to proteins (antibody or other) that inhibit the reaction between a coagulation enzyme and its substrate.

14.4.1 COAGULATION FACTORS

The nomenclature of the coagulation factors is indicated in Table 14–2.

The coagulation process may be divided into several stages. The final phase of coagulation involves the formation of fibrin.

TABLE 14–2.—COAGULATION FACTOR NOMENCLATURE

Factor	
I	Fibrinogen
II	Prothrombin
III	Tissue thromboplastin
IV	Calcium
V	
VII	
VIII	Antihemophilic
IX	Christmas, PTC*
X	Stuart
XI	PTA*
XII	Hageman
XIII	Fibrin-stabilizing

*PTC = thromboplastin component; PTA = thromboplastin antecedent.

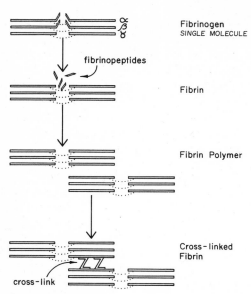

Fig. 14–5.—Steps in cross-linked fibrin formation. α, β and γ are the polypeptide chains of fibrinogen.

14.4.2 FIBRIN FORMATION

Fibrin formation results from the action of the enzyme thrombin on fibrinogen. Thrombin produces limited proteolysis of the fibrinogen molecule, cleaving two small peptides, fibrinopeptides A and B, from the fibrinogen molecule and producing fibrin monomer (Fig. 14–5). Fibrin monomer polymerizes and precipitates out of solution to form the visible clot. Polymerized fibrin is still soluble in acids and in concentrated urea solutions and is hemostatically ineffective. Fibrin polymer is cross-linked by the action of an enzyme, activated factor XIII, which in the presence of calcium forms covalent peptide bonds between the glutamic and lysine amino acids on adjacent molecules. The resulting product is highly insoluble and is hemostatically very effective.

14.4.3 PROTHROMBIN ACTIVATION

Thrombin is formed by the proteolytic cleavage of a proenzyme termed prothrombin. Activation results from the action of activated factor X in the presence of calcium, platelet membrane lipoprotein and factor V (Fig. 14–6).

14.4.4 FACTOR X ACTIVATION

Factor X may be activated by one of two separate pathways. Clinical experience suggests that effective hemostasis requires the participation of both pathways. One pathway is termed the extrinsic system (Fig. 14–7, A). In this process a tissue factor (tissue thromboplastin), released from damaged cells, activates factor X in the presence of factor VII and calcium.

Factor X also can be activated by the intrinsic or "cascade" system (Fig. 14–7, B). The intrinsic pathway is initiated by contact of blood with a "foreign" surface such as collagen or skin, which activates factor XII. Activated factor XII in turn activates factor XI, which, in its turn, in the presence of calcium, activates factor IX. Activated factor IX converts factor X into the activated form in the presence of platelet membrane lipoprotein, factor VIII and calcium. The term

Fig. 14–6.—Prothrombin activation. Prothrombin activator is a complex on the platelet membrane lipoprotein of factor Xa, factor V and calcium ions.

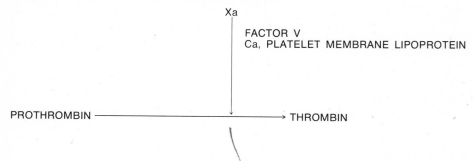

A, EXTRINSIC SYSTEM:

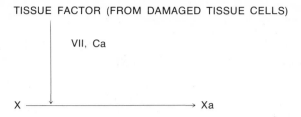

B, INTRINSIC SYSTEM (CASCADE):

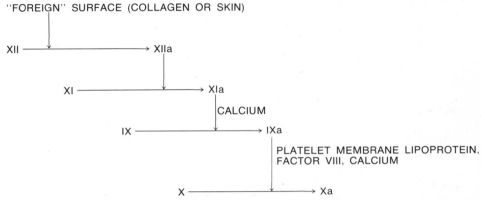

Fig. 14–7.—A, the tissue factor-activated pathway of blood coagulation (extrinsic system). **B,** the surface-activated pathway of blood coagulation (intrinsic system).

cascade was used because it was thought that the intrinsic system acts as an amplifier system. Indeed, if we consider the weight of protein activated at the different stages of the coagulation system, we note that about 0.15 mg of factor VIII leads to the activation of about 1.6 mg of factor X, which subsequently activates about 15 mg of prothrombin, which, in turn, activates about 300 mg of fibrinogen.

14.4.5 TESTS OF THE COAGULATION MECHANISM

The intrinsic pathway of blood coagulation, up to and including fibrin polymerization, is tested by the whole blood clotting time and partial thromboplastin time (Fig. 14–8). The whole blood clotting time tests the time taken for 1 ml of whole blood to clot. The temperature (37 C) and exposure of the blood to the glass surface of the test tube are controlled. The test is influenced by gross defects in the intrinsic clotting system (see Fig. 14–7, B).

The partial thromboplastin time (celite or kaolin-cephalin time) is the time for recalcified citrated plasma to clot. A standardized platelet substitute (cephalin or "partial thromboplastin") and standard surface activation (provided by celite or kaolin) are used to eliminate variability due to the platelet count and surface factors. The test is influenced by moderate defects in the intrinsic clotting system (see Fig. 14–7, B).

The activity of any of the coagulation factors involved in the intrinsic pathway (factors XII, XI, IX and VIII) may be measured by comparing the ability of control and test plasma samples to shorten the partial thromboplastin time of a plasma sample known to be deficient in the specific factor.

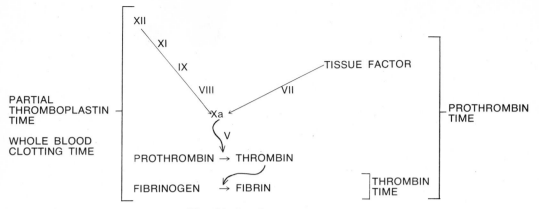

Fig. 14–8.—Coagulation tests.

The extrinsic clotting system is tested by the one-stage prothrombin time. In this test the time taken for recalcified citrated plasma to clot in the presence of tissue thromboplastin is measured. The test is relatively sensitive to defects in the extrinsic clotting system (see Figs. 14–7, A and 14–8). The activity of the extrinsic system coagulation factors (factors II, V, VII and X) may be measured by comparing the ability of control and test plasma samples to shorten the prothrombin time of plasma deficient in the specific factor.

The polymerization of fibrinogen is tested by measuring the thrombin clotting time. This test measures the time for citrated plasma to clot in the presence of added thrombin. The test is abnormal in the presence of heparin or of acquired or congenital abnormalities of the fibrinogen molecule.

14.5 Blood Fluidity System (Regulator Mechanisms)

In addition to the coagulation factors, a complex set of mechanisms exists in the circulation for maintaining the blood in a fluid state. In the absence of this system, sufficient thrombin could be generated by clotting of only 1 ml of blood to coagulate all the fibrinogen in 3 liters of blood. The fluidity-maintaining system consists of both cellular and humoral components.

The cellular component comprises the reticuloendothelial system and liver, which specifically remove activated clotting factors and fibrin without affecting precursor (unactivated) coagulation factors. The humoral component consists of several proteins that specifically inactivate the activated coagulation factors. These proteins include antithrombin and α2-macroglobulin. In addition, the humoral system includes the fibrinolytic mechanism for dissolving fibrin. Fibrinolysis is produced by the action of an enzyme, plasmin, which is itself formed from a precursor, plasminogen (Fig. 14–9). Plasminogen is activated by an extrinsic system (the activator is supplied by damaged cells) and by an intrinsic system, in which the components are all present in the blood. The intrinsic plasmin system is initiated by contact of factor XII with a foreign surface; by way of a number of intermediates, an activator is formed that converts plasminogen to plasmin (see Fig. 14–9). Plasmin attacks peptide bonds involving lysine and not only digests fibrin but also other coagulation factors, including fibrinogen. The polypeptide products of digestion of fibrinogen and fibrin are called fibrinogen/fibrin degradation products (FDP). These degradation products are of various sizes. Some of the larger of these molecular fragments compete with fibrinogen as a substrate for the action of thrombin

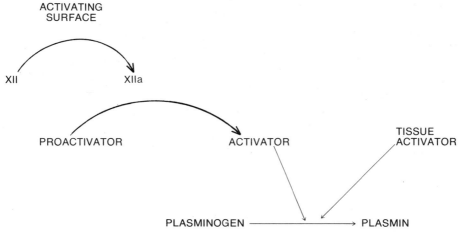

Fig. 14–9.—Activation of plasminogen.

and prolong the thrombin time. FDP also disrupt fibrin polymerization by interposing molecular fragments into the ordered fibrin polymer. Degradation products also inhibit platelet aggregation.

Plasminogen becomes incorporated in the growing clot as fibrin is deposited. This separates plasminogen from the circulating inhibitors of plasminogen activation and permits plasmin formation localized at the site of coagulation. By this mechanism discrete local lysis of fibrin can occur without proteolysis of circulating fibrinogen. Clot lysis following fibrin deposition results in release of fibrin degradation products into the blood. In those pathologic conditions with extensive intravascular clotting, fibrin degradation products may accumulate in the blood without detectable plasmin levels in the blood sampled from a distant site such as an arm vein.

14.6 Production, Distribution, and Life Span of Coagulation Factors

Because all plasma clotting factors except factor VIII are depressed in patients with massive liver necrosis, it is believed that hepatic parenchymal cells make all factors ex-

cept factor VIII. There is evidence that factor VIII antigen is synthesized by endothelial cells, but it is uncertain how factor VIII coagulant activity arises. Factor VIII levels rise sharply after a burst of muscular exercise or an infusion of epinephrine but not on repetition of either stimulus. The rise apparently reflects the release of limited stores of factor VIII into the circulation.

Stress, fever and infection elevate fibrinogen and factor VIII levels by an unknown mechanism. Gram-negative bacterial endotoxin also stimulates fibrinogen production. Factors VII, VIII, X and fibrinogen levels are elevated in pregnancy and in patients using oral contraceptives.

The plasma clotting factors have short intravascular half-lives compared to other plasma proteins. The factors may be grouped in order of decreasing intravascular half-life: (1) fibrinogen, factor XIII – 3 – 5 days; (2) prothrombin, factors V, IX, X, XI, XII – 1 – 3 days; (3) factor VIII – 12 hours and (4) factor VII – 5 hours. Because of these relatively short half-lives, control of postoperative or injury bleeding in a patient with a severe clotting factor deficiency usually requires repeated, daily-to-twice daily replacement therapy during the period of healing.

Disorders of Hemostasis: Diagnostic Approach

15.1 Introduction

THE DIAGNOSIS of coagulation disorders is based on both clinical and laboratory evidence. A careful and knowledgeably collected history is essential if the results of laboratory studies are to be properly interpreted.

15.2 The History

A history taken to evaluate hemostasis should answer the following questions:

1. Has there been abnormal bleeding or bruising either spontaneously or after injury, dental extraction or surgery?

2. Was bleeding delayed and prolonged following the injury, suggesting a coagulation disorder, or immediate and transient, suggesting a platelet disorder?

3. Was there bleeding from the umbilical stump?

4. Was there excessive bleeding after circumcision?

5. Was there, during childhood, excessive bleeding from cuts in the mouth?

The central incisors have erupted by the time most infants are learning to walk; many children fall and cut their lips and gums at this time.

6. What are the frequency and size of hematomas of the scalp?

7. What was the extent of bruising from minor trauma, e.g., falls from swings, from bicycles or down steps?

8. Are there prolonged nose bleeds? Brief epistaxis that stops within minutes, even if frequent, is usually associated with normal tests of hemostasis.

In adult patients, an attempt should be made to determine the degree and frequency of the following:

1. Bruising. Spontaneous bruises larger than the palm of the hand are generally significant; a history of hematomas and bruises at the sites of injections or immunizations may likewise be revealing.

2. Excessive bleeding from small cuts. Specific details as to size of laceration and duration of bleeding should be elicited.

3. Bleeding after previous surgery. Pa-

tients readily recall major surgery; they often need prompting to recall minor procedures.

4. Other disorder. Does the patient show evidence of an acquired disorder that may be accompanied by a hemostatic disorder, such as liver disease, SLE, uremia or a hematologic malignancy?

5. Medication. Is the patient taking medication that may interfere with hemostasis?

6. Family history of bleeding. If present, what is the hereditary pattern of transmission?

In questioning a parent about bleeding in a small child, inquiry should be made about the following:

1. Bleeding during or immediately after surgery. This may be entirely normal, but late bleeding, e.g., bleeding beginning on the third postoperative day, is more suggestive of a hemostatic disorder.

2. Bleeding after dental extractions. Many small blood vessels are torn during extraction of a permanent tooth, providing a good test of hemostasis. Postextraction bleeding lasting longer than 24 hours, or fresh bleeding after 3 or 4 days, should arouse suspicion of abnormal hemostasis. A history of extractions without abnormal bleeding weighs against a hereditary bleeding tendency.

Drugs that interfere with hemostasis fall into two categories:

1. Drugs that impair formation of the hemostatic plug. Aspirin, in ordinary doses, can prolong bleeding time and should be discontinued several days before surgery. Other drugs that interfere with platelet function include dipyridamole, clofibrate, phenylbutazone, antihistamines and tranquilizers. However, the clinical significance of these drugs with respect to hemostasis has yet to be clearly documented.

2. Drugs that interfere with blood clotting, including heparin and the oral coumarin drugs. Although preoperative patients are rarely receiving parenteral heparin, patients will be encountered who are receiving long-term oral anticoagulant therapy.

15.3 Physical Examination

Evidence of the following should be sought:

1. Abnormal bleeding in the skin. Ecchymoses suggest abnormal bleeding from relatively large vessels due to a defect in blood clotting. Petechiae, which may be small, require a careful search, particularly around the ankles, as they suggest increased vascular fragility secondary to thrombocytopenia.

2. Mucosal bleeding. Purpura of the buccal mucosa and the conjunctival surfaces of the eyelids should be sought. Hemorrhagic bullae in the mouth are found only in the presence of thrombocytopenia. Hemorrhages in the optic fundi, however, may reflect local ocular pathology, hypertension, diabetes, severe anemia or thrombocytopenia.

3. Hereditary connective tissue disorder. Abnormal elasticity of the skin and hyperextensibility of the joints may be associated with vascular bleeding.

4. Chronic liver diseases. Signs include spider angiomas, palmar erythema, dilated abdominal veins, hepatomegaly or splenomegaly.

15.4 Laboratory Studies

A careful history is the best screening test available. Nevertheless, laboratory screening tests for the integrity of coagulation and platelet components of the hemostatic mechanism are indicated under a number of circumstances, including:

1. Historical or physical evidence of abnormal hemostasis.

2. Family history of abnormal hemostasis.

3. Presence of a disease that may be associated with abnormal hemostasis, e.g., liver failure, SLE.

4. Prior to surgical procedures known to be associated with a high incidence of hemorrhage.

15.4.1 COAGULATION SYSTEM

A commonly used set of screening tests includes (1) prothrombin time, (2) partial thromboplastin time, (3) thrombin clotting time and (4) fibrinogen concentration; most tests of fibrinogen depend on measuring the concentration of thrombin-clottable protein in the plasma.

If one or more of these coagulation system screening tests are abnormal, then, based on the history and any abnormal tests, an assessment is made as to the probable defect. The factor(s) most likely to be abnormal should be specifically assayed, including factor XIII.

If all coagulation system screening tests are normal, no further tests are necessary unless there is a history very strongly suggestive of abnormal hemostasis.

15.4.2 PLATELET SYSTEM

Basic screening tests include (1) bleeding time and (2) platelet count.

Tests that screen for defects of platelet function include (1) clot retraction, (2) platelet factor 3 activity and (3) platelet aggregation.

If bleeding time is prolonged and thrombocytopenia is detected, the etiology of the thrombocytopenia should be pursued, including a careful history for exposure to drugs or toxins, physical examination for splenomegaly and systemic disease, a complete blood count, examination of bone marrow and tests for SLE and antibodies to platelets.

If the bleeding time is prolonged and the platelet count is normal, tests for von Willebrand's disease and for platelet function should be undertaken.

Vascular Defects

16.1 Clinical Features

VASCULAR DEFECTS (non-thrombocytopenic purpuras) are common but they usually do not cause a serious bleeding problem. Bleeding mainly occurs from mucous membranes or into the skin. Bleeding starts immediately following injury, ceases in less than 24–48 hours and rarely recurs. The mechanism of bleeding is thought to be damage to capillary endothelium. The platelet count usually is normal, but tests of platelet function may be normal or abnormal. In patients in whom a platelet function defect is demonstrable, the actual role of the vascular defect in the pathogenesis of the bleeding syndrome is uncertain and there is no current method for diagnosing the vascular defect under such circumstances. In many cases the diagnosis of a vascular defect underlying the bleeding syndrome is by exclusion. The platelet count and bleeding time usually are normal. A number of disease syndromes may be accompanied by bleeding thought to be due to vascular defects.

16.1.1 INFECTIONS

Many severe infections may be associated with bleeding manifestations, especially typhoid fever, subacute bacterial endocarditis, meningococcemia, septicemia and sometimes childhood viral infections such as measles. Disorders of platelet function, thrombocytopenia and coagulation (defibrination) as well as vascular defects may play a role.

16.1.2 IMPLICATION OF DRUGS

In addition to the purpura, some other type of rash, often urticarial or maculopapular, may be present. Examples of drugs that may be associated with purpura include penicillin and the sulfonamides.

16.1.3 SCURVY

This nutritional disorder involving deficiency of vitamin C is very rare in the U. S. The pathogenic mechanism in scurvy is defective intercellular substance of capillary walls. There is a failure in collagen formation associated with defective hydroxyproline synthesis. Hydroxyproline is not synthesized in the absence of ascorbic acid. In addition, a defect of platelet function has been described in some cases of scurvy. Bleeding may occur in the skin, characteristically perifollicular; in the muscles, particularly the calf muscles; in the gastrointestinal tract or into the urine. Clinical signs that suggest scurvy are swelling of the gums and hyperkeratosis of the skin. If a diagnosis is suspected, it can be confirmed by demonstrating a low WBC ascorbic acid content. Treatment is administration of vitamin C.

16.1.4 THE CUSHING SYNDROME

The basic pathologic defect in this disorder, characterized by excessive cortisol production, is thought to be the protein-wasting effect of the increased blood steroid level. However, the effect must be complex because there is clinical evidence that pharmacologic administration of steroids decreases the bleeding associated with thrombocytopenia.

16.1.5 HENOCH-SCHÖNLEIN SYNDROME

Also known as anaphylactoid purpura or hypersensitivity angiitis, this relatively uncommon disorder is thought to be a hypersensitivity reaction related to acute nephritis and rheumatic fever. Pathologically, an acute inflammatory reaction of the capillaries and mesangial tissues of the small arterioles is found associated with increased vascular permeability, exudation and hemorrhage into the tissues. Food, drugs and bacteria have been implicated in hypersensitivity angiitis without definitive evidence for any of these. The syndrome is most common in children, usually preceded by streptococcal sore throat 1–3 weeks before the onset of hemorrhagic manifestations. The clinical pattern includes the following:

1. Purpuric rash. Purpuric spots may be small or large. Initially they may be urticarial and they often have a characteristic distribution on the extensor surfaces of the arms, legs and buttocks. The character and distribution of the rash may be the only clue as to the diagnosis of the syndrome.

2. Abdominal manifestations, e.g., colicky pain due to extravasation of fluid and blood into the intestinal wall.

3. Polyarthralgia and polyarthritis.

4. Hematuria, often with albuminuria, casts and the clinical spectrum of acute diffuse glomerulonephritis, including edema and hypertension. The vast majority of patients recover completely, but an occasional patient may die in acute renal failure or develop chronic nephritis. Tests of platelet function and coagulation are normal.

16.1.6 SENILE PURPURA

This condition occurs most commonly in thin elderly people and usually affects the extensor surfaces of the arms. Irregular, dark purple areas with clear-cut margins are present on the arms, and the skin is freely mobile over the deeper tissues. The disorder is thought to be due to atrophy of collagen so that the skin is not well anchored to deeper tissues and movements easily rupture vessels.

16.1.7 HEREDITARY HEMORRHAGIC TELANGIECTASIA

This syndrome is transmitted as a simple dominant trait affecting both sexes equally. The telangiectases are due to multiple dilatations of capillaries and arterioles, which are lined by a thin layer of endothelial cells. The bleeding tendency is thought to be due to mechanical fragility of the dilated vessel. Clinically, the telangiectases may be on any part of the skin as well as on the mucosae of the nose and mouth, gastrointestinal tract or renal tract. Bleeding may occur from any one of these sites and in a recurrent fashion. Telangiectases present on the skin blanch on pressure, since the blood is not extravascular but within the capillary dilatation. The diagnosis is made from the clinical triad of telangiectasis, hemorrhage and familial pattern.

17

Platelet Disorders

17.1 Introduction

PLATELET DISORDERS may be due to an altered number or altered function of the platelets. Disorders of platelet number include thrombocytopenia (platelet count too low) and thrombocythemia or thrombocytosis (platelet count too high). There are many disorders of platelet function, and the terms thrombasthenia (a severe functional defect) and thrombocytopathy (a milder functional defect) are frequently used.

17.2 Mechanisms of Thrombocytopenia

The most common serious bleeding disorder involving platelets is thrombocytopenia.

Too low a platelet count may result from any one or a combination of mechanisms. These include decreased platelet production, disordered platelet distribution and increased rate of platelet destruction (Table 17–1).

Disordered production of platelets may result from decreased production or defective maturation. When platelet production is significantly decreased, the number of megakaryocytes visible in a bone marrow aspirate usually is significantly decreased.

Decreased production of platelets may result from (1) administration of drugs such as cytotoxic agents used in cancer chemotherapy (the most common cause of thrombocytopenia in a large medical center), gold, sulfonamides and ethanol; (2) irradiation of bone marrow; (3) generalized decrease in

TABLE 17–1.—CAUSES OF THROMBOCYTOPENIA

Production Defect
  Reduced production
    Marrow injury: drugs, chemicals, radiation, infection
    Marrow failure: acquired, congenital
    Marrow invasion: carcinoma, leukemia, lymphoma, fibrosis
  Ineffective thrombopoiesis
  B_{12} deficiency
  Folate deficiency
  Hereditary
Sequestration
  Splenomegaly
  Hypothermic anesthesia
Accelerated Destruction
  Antibodies
    Autoantibodies
      ITP, SLE, hemolytic anemias, lymphoreticular disorders
      Drugs: quinidine, quinine, sedormid
    Alloantibodies
      Fetal-maternal incompatibility
      Following transfusions
  Nonimmunologic
    Disseminated intravascular coagulation
    Infections
    Prosthetic cardiac valves
    Thrombotic thrombocytopenic purpura
    Other, e.g., massive transfusion, ristocetin

production of all marrow cells (aplastic anemia; see Chapter 3); (4) marrow replacement or infiltration (myelophthisis) including marrow fibrosis, leukemia and metastatic carcinoma and (5) maturation disorders, i.e., bone marrow shows a normal or increased number of megakaryocytes, but thrombopoiesis is ineffective in a manner analogous to ineffective erythropoiesis. Diseases associated with disordered maturation include (1) vitamin B_{12} or folate deficiency (see section 5.2) and (2) the myeloproliferative disorders (see Chapter 11).

Disordered distribution of platelets may be the cause of thrombocytopenia. As previously mentioned, in normal individuals about 20% of the circulating platelets at any one time are present in the spleen. With massive splenomegaly, up to 80% of the total number of circulating platelets may be in the spleen, resulting in peripheral blood thrombocytopenia.

Increased destruction of platelets is a frequent cause of thrombocytopenia. The survival time of platelets is markedly decreased from the normal 10 days to less than 1 day. The commonest causes of accelerated platelet destruction are antibody-mediated platelet injury, increased platelet utilization in disseminated intravascular coagulation (DIC), and massive blood transfusion.

Antibody-mediated thrombocytopenias may be due to the following:

1. *Autoantibodies* in such disorders as idiopathic thrombocytopenic purpura (ITP; see section 17.4), SLE (see section 17.5.2) and chronic lymphocytic leukemia, and in association with autoimmune hemolytic anemia (see section 17.5.2).

2. *Alloantibodies* associated with pregnancy or transfusion.

3. *Antibodies* associated with use of drugs such as quinidine, quinine and sulfonamides (see section 17.5.1).

Increased in vivo thrombin occurs in conditions that produce *DIC* (see section 18.2.5); under these conditions thrombocytopenia may develop due to an increased rate of destruction of platelets.

Following *massive transfusion* of blood, thrombocytopenia may occur due to (1) dilution with platelet-depleted stored blood, or (2) the presence of antiplatelet antibodies in transfused blood.

17.3 Clinical Considerations in Thrombocytopenia

The normal platelet count ranges from 150,000–400,000/cu mm. Thrombocytopenia is generally considered to be present when the platelet count is less than 100,000/cu mm. There is a rough relationship between the platelet count and severity of bleeding. With platelet counts above 40,000/cu mm, bleeding may occur after accidental injury or surgery, but spontaneous bleeding is uncommon. Spontaneous bleeding is common with platelet counts between 10,000/cu mm and 40,000/cu mm; with counts below

20,000/cu mm it is usual and often severe.

Spontaneous bleeding may be present on the skin in the form of petechiae, purpuric spots or confluent ecchymoses. In the mouth, petechiae or blood-filled bullae are almost always pathognomonic of thrombocytopenia. Bleeding may occur from any mucous membrane including the nose and uterus and gastrointestinal, urinary and respiratory tracts. The most serious site for spontaneous bleeding is the central nervous system, where hemorrhage may be fatal. Bleeding due to trauma to a thrombocytopenic patient presents a number of features distinct from those of a patient with a coagulation factor disorder: (1) it occurs immediately after the trauma; (2) in mild cases it may cease in response to local pressure and (3) in any case bleeding usually stops within 48 hours and does not readily recur.

17.4 Idiopathic Thrombocytopenic Purpura

17.4.1 CLINICAL FEATURES

ITP may be considered the prototype thrombocytopenic disorder. The chief symptom is purpura on the arms, legs, upper chest and neck. Mucosal bleeding may occur. There usually is no fever or malaise. Physical examination shows no adenopathy and the spleen is not palpable in 90% of patients; when palpable, the spleen usually does not extend more than 1 cm below the left costal margin.

The course of ITP may be acute or chronic. The acute form of the disease occurs most commonly in children but it is seen in adults as well. There is a sudden onset of bleeding, usually most severe initially and ceasing within a few days. The risk of cerebral hemorrhage is greatest in the first 2 weeks. Some patients may display the bleeding tendency for several months but most stop bleeding within 6 months; occasionally bleeding persists and becomes chronic. The chronic re-

current form of ITP occurs most often in women between 20 and 40 years of age. Onset is usually more gradual and intermittent than in the acute form. Transient remissions are characteristic and may last weeks, months or years.

It should be remembered that ITP may present with bleeding localized to one site only, e.g., menorrhagia, hematuria or epistaxis. In such patients, ITP should be suspected and a bleeding time and platelet count should be done.

17.4.2 LABORATORY TESTS

A low platelet count is present in the peripheral blood smear and the platelets are normal morphologically; large, atypical forms may occasionally be present. The bleeding time is prolonged proportional to the degree of thrombocytopenia. The whole blood clotting time test is normal but clot retraction is poor or absent when the platelet count is below 40,000/cu mm. Anemia is present only to the extent of blood loss and the erythrocyte sedimentation rate usually is normal. Bone marrow examination reveals megakaryocytes in normal or increased numbers, with normal morphology.

17.4.3 DIAGNOSIS

A significant degree of splenomegaly suggests another diagnosis, as also does the presence of fever, disproportionate anemia or a high sedimentation rate. Bone marrow aspiration is essential to exclude other marrow diseases; the spleen should be examined histologically for the same reason, if it is removed for therapeutic reasons. It is important to exclude other diagnoses, in particular drug-induced thrombocytopenia on a sensitization basis. This is very important, because the clinical and hematologic pictures of ITP and drug-induced hypersensitivity thrombocytopenic purpura are indistinguishable from a hematologic point of view. A careful history is the only clue to the possibility of drug-induced thrombocytopenia. SLE and other diseases associated with platelet antibodies should be considered, and appropriate serologic tests for SLE should be done in all patients. When thrombocytopenia is due to platelet sequestration in a large spleen, anemia and leukopenia usually are associated. In leukemia, disproportionate anemia is frequent and the marrow is diagnostic. In aplastic anemia, pancytopenia is characteristic and bone marrow biopsy should reveal hypocellularity. In patients with bone marrow infiltration, anemia usually is present, normoblasts and myelocytes are found in the peripheral blood and, again, the marrow is diagnostic.

17.4.4 Pathogenesis

Antiplatelet antibody is present in the plasma of most patients with ITP and can be demonstrated in vitro. Transfusion of plasma from patients with this disease causes transient thrombocytopenia and clinical purpura in the recipient. It also is known that transient thrombocytopenia may occur in infants born to mothers with ITP, suggesting transplacental passage of the antiplatelet factor. The antibody has been shown to be an IgG that sensitizes platelets for sequestration by the spleen and liver. Following splenectomy the liver may become the chief site for sequestration. The term autoimmune thrombocytopenic purpura has been suggested as an alternative name for ITP.

17.4.5 Treatment of Acute ITP

The majority of patients, frequently children, with acute ITP will recover in time regardless of therapy; hence conservative management is favored, as follows:

1. *Corticosteroids* do not appear to shorten the duration of thrombocytopenia, but 1–2 mg/kg/day of prednisone is advisable during the first 2 weeks because of the beneficial effect on capillary integrity.

2. *Platelet transfusions* may be of transient benefit in treating severe hemorrhage.

3. About 20% of children with ITP fail to recover in 6 months and their course is similar to that of adults with chronic ITP (see section 17.4.6). About 30% have no or mild symptoms and do not require therapy. The remaining 50% generally can be controlled with *prednisone*. Since growth retardation and steroid complications may occur, *splenectomy* is usually advised if steroids are required beyond 3–6 months. Splenectomy carried out on such patients is beneficial in 85%.

4. *Immunosuppressive therapy* may be considered if splenectomy fails.

17.4.6 Treatment of Chronic ITP

1. *Platelet transfusion* is often effective in treating life-threatening hemorrhage but should not be used prophylactically because of the short platelet lifespan and because of isoantibody formation.

2. *Adrenocortical steroids* produce a beneficial effect by suppressing the phagocytic activity of the reticuloendothelial system and improving the life span of antibody-coated platelets. A dose of 0.5 mg/kg/day of prednisone will elevate the platelet count in mild cases of intermediate severity; and 2 mg or more/kg/day may be necessary if the platelet count is less than 10,000/cu mm. The platelet count usually does not rise for several days and often not for up to 14 days. The majority of patients will show an elevation of platelet level in response to steroids. If improvement does not occur within 2–3 weeks or can be maintained only with massive doses of steroids, the spleen should be removed. In patients who respond to steroids, dosage should be gradually reduced over a several-week period until the platelet count is about 60,000/cu mm. Splenectomy is favored in patients who fail to recover spontaneously within 1–6 months, who require more than 5–10 mg/day of prednisone and who are suitable operative risks.

3. *Splenectomy* removes the major site of platelet destruction. The prednisone dosage

should be increased to raise the platelet count prior to surgery. Platelet transfusion may be used in the presence of severe thrombocytopenia but usually is not required in the less severe cases. After splenectomy 80% of patients improve, and the platelet count is restored to normal levels permanently in 66%. The count may rise within 24 hours or within a week of surgery. There is no certain method of predicting a successful response to splenectomy. Following splenectomy steroids should be withdrawn gradually over a 3-week period. If steroids are still required to prevent purpura or severe thrombocytopenia, immunosuppression should be considered.

4. *Immunosuppression,* e.g., use of azathioprine, cyclophosphamide or vincristine, may be beneficial to patients in whom splenectomy has failed. An approximate 50–70% response to each of these drugs has been reported.

17.5 Secondary Thrombocytopenia

By this term is meant thrombocytopenia in association with a known cause or a primary disease (see Table 17–1). In each of these conditions the first principle of therapy is direction of specific measures at the established cause. Adrenocortical steroids may lessen bleeding, but results are not as good as in ITP.

17.5.1 Thrombocytopenia Due to Drugs and Chemicals

Thrombocytopenia due to drugs and chemicals may be part of the marrow depression that occurs with cytotoxic agents used in therapy of leukemia, lymphoma and carcinoma. Generalized marrow depression and consequent pancytopenia also may occur with other drugs such as gold or the sulfonamides. Thrombocytopenia also may result from a specific effect on the megakaryocytes or as a part of a hypersensitivity reaction. In such cases selective thrombocytopenia occurs. The drug is thought to bind to a plasma protein to form the primary antigen. Antibodies stimulated by the primary antigen bind the drug, and thrombocytopenia occurs when drug-antibody complexes form, with a high affinity for the platelet membrane. The drugs most commonly associated with hypersensitivity reactions are quinidine, quinine and sedormid.

The clinical manifestation of thrombocytopenia, associated with ingestion of a drug to which the individual is hypersensitive, is bleeding, and this often occurs within hours or days of drug administration. In other patients bleeding may occur after months, weeks or days of ingestion of the drug. Bleeding is often severe and sudden in onset and may be associated with fever and systemic symptoms.

Thrombocytopenia is present and the bone marrow may show either increased numbers of megakaryocytes when peripheral blood destruction of platelets is the mechanism (hypersensitivity reactions) or a reduced number of megakaryocytes and other marrow elements (marrow depression). Evidence of drug hypersensitivity may be demonstrable in vitro. The drug may inhibit clot retraction when added to the patient's blood, but this test is relatively insensitive. The most sensitive test for drug hypersensitivity is a complement fixation test.

Hypersensitivity thrombocytopenia generally responds briskly to withdrawal of the offending drug, and, therefore, therapy includes immediate withdrawal of implicated drugs. The patient should be given a card indicating the drug sensitivity. Adrenocorticosteroids and platelet transfusions should be given for control of bleeding. Splenectomy is not indicated. When thrombocytopenia is part of aplastic anemia, the prognosis is that of the aplastic anemia.

17.5.2 THROMBOCYTOPENIA AND HEMOLYTIC ANEMIA WITH FRAGMENTED RED CELLS

Disorders that display the combination of thrombocytopenia and hemolysis with fragmented red cells (see Fig. 2–2, G) include:

1. *Thrombotic thrombocytopenic purpura,* a fulminating, generally lethal disorder characterized by hemolytic anemia with severely fragmented red cells, thrombocytopenic purpura, fever, renal failure and fluctuating, often bizarre neurologic manifestations. The typical pathologic lesion consists of widespread hyaline occlusions of small vessels. The etiology and pathogenesis of the disorder are unknown. There is no established therapy, but large doses of prednisone and emergency splenectomy have been associated with recovery in some patients.

2. *SLE,* in which thrombocytopenia usually results from a platelet autoantibody and hemolysis from a red cell autoantibody. In an occasional patient fragmented red cells may be present, possibly resulting from mechanical red cell damage due to contact with fibrin deposited in vessels.

3. *Neoplasms,* which may be obvious, with widespread metastases, or occult. Diffuse intravascular clotting-accelerated catabolism of platelets and anemia with fragmented red cells may be associated.

4. *Hemolytic-uremia syndromes.* In infants and small children, fever, acute hemolysis with fragmented red cells, thrombocytopenia and renal failure may occur. An occasional patient has evidence of DIC and may respond favorably to heparin therapy. The pathogenic mechanism in these patients, without evidence of intravascular coagulation, is unclear. Hemolysis with fragmented red cells and thrombocytopenia may occur as a complication of pregnancy or the puerperium when toxemia is present. The pathogenic mechanism is not established.

17.6 Platelet Transfusions

Platelet transfusions are useful in preventing or stopping bleeding due to thrombocytopenia. Platelets should be transfused within about 6 hours of collection since they lose viability rapidly after that time. Generally in adults transfusions involving about 8–15 units of platelet concentrate are used and elevate the platelet count temporarily above 30,000/cu mm.

Repeated platelet transfusion can result in isoimmunization and failure of response to further infusion. Following isoimmunization there may be a satisfactory response to HL-A-compatible platelets but these may be very difficult to obtain. In view of this, platelet transfusions are restricted to therapy of life-threatening or serious hemorrhage and to tide a patient over an acute period of severe thrombocytopenia of less than 10,000/cu mm. Conditions in which platelet transfusions may be used, based on these principles, include (1) acute leukemia, (2) aplastic anemia with serious hemorrhage, (3) acute idiopathic thrombocytopenia manifesting serious bleeding, (4) exsanguinating blood loss requiring massive blood transfusion and (5) uremia with bleeding prior to dialysis.

17.7 Thrombocytosis and Thrombocythemia

Thrombocytosis is a temporary elevation of platelet count that may occur after severe hemorrhage, surgery and splenectomy and in iron deficiency. Thrombocytosis may be associated with a tendency to thrombosis. The term *thrombocythemia* refers to a sustained elevation of platelet count, usually above 800,000/cu mm. In this condition, generally considered to be a variant of the myeloproliferative disorders, the spleen almost always is palpably enlarged. Conditions associated with thrombocythemia include polycythemia vera, chronic myelogenous leukemia and myelosclerosis. When not a part of one of these syndromes, the disorder is termed essential (hemorrhagic) thrombocythemia. Patients with essential thrombocythemia may demonstrate spontaneous bleeding as well as venous and arterial thromboses. Treatment of primary thrombocythemia involves measures to decrease the autonomous growth of megakaryocytes and the excessive platelet production. This therapy involves ^{32}P or busulfan administration. Use of heparin is required if thrombosis de-

velops. The prognosis of primary thrombocythemia is that of the basic myeloproliferative disorder.

17.8 Functional Disorders of Platelets

17.8.1 Congenital

These disorders generally are referred to
by the term *thrombocytopathy*. They usually
present as a mild bleeding tendency. Laboratory manifestations include a slightly prolonged bleeding time, normal platelet count
and normal clot retraction. One or more tests
of platelet function are defective, such as
platelet aggregation in response to ADP,
collagen or norepinephrine. Some patients
have defective quantities of ADP in the
storage granules of platelets, termed *storage
pool disease*. In others, the defect appears to
be a defect of the platelet release reaction,
and ADP content of the storage granules
is normal.

A rare congenital disorder of platelet function is termed *thrombasthenia*. This is associated with a severe hemorrhagic diathesis
with a markedly prolonged bleeding time,
absent clot retraction and absent platelet
aggregation in response to ADP or collagen.

17.8.2 Acquired

Acquired disorders of platelet function
include injury due to drugs, the most common being aspirin and phenylbutazone.
The aspirin effect is mediated by inhibition
of cyclo-oxygenase production of prostaglandin cyclic endoperoxides. Other anti-
inflammatory drugs may impair platelet function by inhibiting the platelet release reaction.
Analgesic drugs that do not impair platelet
function include acetaminophen and propoxyphene. *Uremia* with marked nitrogen
retention may be associated with generalized bleeding from mucosal surfaces as
well as cutaneous bleeding due to a platelet
defect. This defect in platelet function is
rapidly reversed by dialysis.

Certain *dysproteinemias* may be associated with a defect of platelet function. In patients with macroglobulinemia or myeloma,
the abnormal globulin is thought to coat the
platelet and interfere with its proper function. In *benign hyperglobulinemic purpura*,
purpuric spots are found characteristically
on the anterior aspects of the lower limbs in
association with an elevated gamma globulin
level in the serum. The pathogenesis of this
disorder is unknown.

18

Disorders of Coagulation

18.1 Congenital Coagulation Disorders

THESE RELATIVELY RARE DISORDERS usually reflect defects in the activity of single coagulation factors. Rarely, two or more factors may be defective in the same patient.

18.1.1 HEMOPHILIA

Hemophilia is due to an inherited deficiency in the activity of the antihemophilic globulin, factor VIII. It is the most common of the congenital coagulation factor disorders, with an incidence of about one in 10,000 of the population. The gene is transmitted in a sex-linked recessive pattern (Fig. 18–1). Female heterozygotes (carriers) transmit the disorder to one half of their sons, and the gene to one half of their daughters. Female carriers generally do not manifest any bleeding tendency. The measured level of factor VIII cannot absolutely establish whether the sister of a hemophilic male is a carrier (heterozygote) or is normal. If the sister has a factor VIII level of 60% or less, she has a greater than 90% chance of being heterozygous for the hemophilic gene. If she has a factor VIII level of 100% or greater, she has an 80% chance of being free of the mutant gene. Males with the disorder (hemizygotes) transmit the gene to all daughters; all sons are normal. In 30% of patients, no family history can be detected.

18.1.1.1 NATURE OF THE DEFECT.—Recently there has been intense interest in the biochemistry of the factor VIII molecule. Several independently isolated factor VIII preparations have a molecular weight of about 1.1 million and a similar amino acid

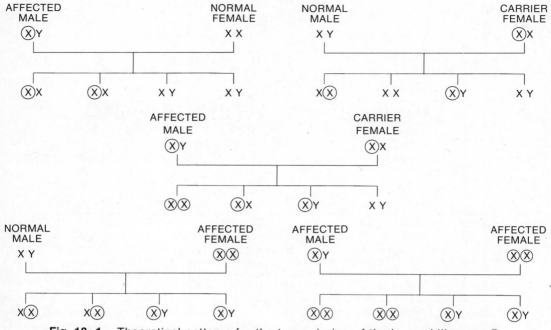

Fig. 18—1.—Theoretical patterns for the transmission of the hemophilia gene ⊗.

composition. Antibodies to these preparations have been developed. The plasma of hemophilic patients has normal amounts of the factor VIII antigen recognized by these antibodies.

At the present time, the factor VIII antigen is often referred to as factor VIII-related protein or as factor VIII. In the presence of calcium chloride or high salt concentration, this factor VIII-related protein dissociates into a small molecular weight fraction, which has factor VIII-coagulant activity, and a large molecular weight fraction, is devoid of coagulant activity but carries the factor VIII-related protein antigenic specificity. A definitive interpretation of these data is not possible at present, but it may be that the smaller moiety is the true factor VIII-coagulant molecule and the larger molecule a factor VIII transport or binding protein, or alternatively that the smaller fraction is derived from the larger by proteolysis.

18.1.1.2 CLINICAL FEATURES. — In severely affected patients the disorder presents itself in infancy. In milder cases it may not be manifest until later in life and only at the time of an injury. The severity of clinical manifestations is closely related to the degree of deficiency in factor VIII activity (Table 18 – 1). The clinical course is characterized by unpredictable fluctuations in the severity of the bleeding tendency. Bleeding is characteristically slow and persists for days or weeks, despite the formation of large friable clots. The onset is delayed hours or days after the actual injury. Recurrent bleeding is particularly common. Bleeding may occur anywhere, and deep tissue bleeding may vary from a few milliliters to liters of blood. Bruising of the skin may occur, but not petechiae. Lacerations and contusions often cause prolonged and troublesome bleeding. The mouth, nose, tongue and frenum of the upper lip are common bleeding sites in children. After tooth extraction, gum sockets almost invariably bleed excessively. In severe cases epistaxis and bleeding into the muscular tissues of the tongue may occur.

TABLE 18-1.—RELATIONSHIP OF
BLOOD LEVELS OF FACTOR VIII
TO SEVERITY OF BLEEDING
MANIFESTATION

BLOOD LEVEL OF FACTOR VIII (% NORMAL)	TYPE OF BLEEDING
50–100	None
25–50	May bleed excessively after major trauma
5–25	Severe bleeding after surgical operations and some bleeding after minor trauma; no spontaneous bleeding
1–5	Severe bleeding after minor injury; occasional spontaneous hemorrhages
0	Severe hemophilia with spontaneous bleeding into muscles and joints

Bleeding into synovial joints is common in severe hemophilia, is less common in moderate hemophilia and may never occur in mild forms of the disorder. Joint bleeding may occur spontaneously or following injury and, although the acute symptoms may last only 3 or 4 days, full recovery may take several weeks. The joints most often affected are ankles, knees and elbows. Chronic arthritis frequently develops in a joint subjected to repeated episodes of bleeding. Permanent joint damage frequently occurs, with destruction of the edge of the bones forming the joints. Osteophytes also may form and lead to limitation of joint movement. Fibrous or bony ankylosis may occur, and contractures of the surrounding muscles may develop.

A chronic hematoma in relation to bone may result in the development of a cystic mass, termed a pseudotumor. Pseudotumors occur most frequently in relation to the pelvic bones or femora. Bleeding into muscles and connective tissue occurs commonly in the limbs. When a limb vessel is occluded by the pressure of the hematoma, ischemic necrosis may occur and result in muscle contracture (Volkmann's contracture).

Bleeding from the gastrointestinal tract is most often the result of associated peptic ulcer. An acute hematoma in the wall of the gut may result in transient gastrointestinal obstruction. Retroperitoneal bleeding may mimic acute appendicitis.

Intracranial bleeding occurs extra- or intracerebrally and is a common cause of death in patients with severe hemophilia. When the hematoma occurs in relation to a specific nerve, acute nerve palsy results. Bleeding into the urogenital tract most commonly presents as hematuria, a common manifestation of hemophilia. Ureteral colic is caused by passage of clots from bleeding from any part of the kidney or ureter. Potentially lethal complications include acute respiratory obstruction by hematomas in the lingual and laryngeal areas, cardiac tamponade due to hematoma in the pericardial cavity and respiratory failure due to bleeding into the pleural cavity.

The excessive bleeding of hemophilia may lead to acute or chronic anemia. Hematomas often are associated with fever and malaise, and the products of heme degradation within resolving hematomas may produce hyperbilirubinemia.

18.1.1.3 DIAGNOSIS.—Hemophilia should be suspected from the clinical and hereditary features of the disease. Suggestive clinical features are the sex of the patient, the familial pattern if present, age at onset and the type of bleeding. A family tree should be drawn while the history is taken. The diagnosis is established by laboratory tests. Tests of platelet function, bleeding time and platelet count are normal. Tests of coagulation show a prolonged whole blood clotting time in severe hemophilia; the clotting time may be normal in mild hemophilia. The one-stage prothrombin time is normal and the partial thromboplastin time is prolonged. A low factor VIII coagulant activity is diagnostic.

18.1.1.4 MANAGEMENT.—Drugs that interfere with platelet function, such as aspirin, should be scrupulously avoided. The hemophilic patient, despite his coagulation defect, has a normal bleeding time, because ADP released from platelets initiates formation of a temporary hemostatic plug. Aspirin interferes with the ADP release reaction, inhibits formation of the hemostatic plug and seriously increases the hazard of bleeding. Acetaminophen or propoxyphene may be used for analgesia without prolongation of the bleeding time.

Intramuscular injections should be avoided in the hemophiliac. Indeed, any patient with a bleeding tendency who needs medication should receive it either orally or intravenously. Intramuscular injections result in large and painful hematomas. Subcutaneous immunization should be given carefully to hemophilic infants and usually does not cause serious bleeding.

Hemophiliacs are in particular need of careful and regular prophylactic dental care. Regular visits to the dentist and prompt filling of cavities may prevent unnecessary extractions.

In the management of patients with hemophilia, it is necessary to consider the patient's life as a whole. The family is in need of help and advice in planning education, in career training, in maintaining physical fitness without injury and in organizing a healthy social life for the affected child. The patient may be advised to join the Hemophilia Society, where he may turn for advice and support. He should carry a card stating his diagnosis and blood group.

Bleeding episodes in the hemophiliac require special measures carefully tailored to the nature of the bleeding and the deficit in coagulation. For minor bleeding local applications of thrombin or epinephrine packs can be helpful. For more significant bleeding, transfusion of factor VIII concentrate is required. The most widely used preparation is a lyophilized cryoprecipitate that contains partially purified factor VIII activity. It is advisable to give infusions at 12-hour intervals (Fig. 18–2; Table 18–2). The amount of factor VIII given depends on the factor VIII level required to provide hemostasis. In patients undergoing surgery, factor VIII levels should be elevated to above 50% of the normal level and maintained above 30% until the wound has healed completely. Prophylactic factor VIII infusion should be given for tooth extraction. Factor VIII levels, approximately half those required for

Fig. 18–2.—Blood levels of factor VIII following a single plasma transfusion in a patient with hemophilia and in one with von Willebrand's disease.

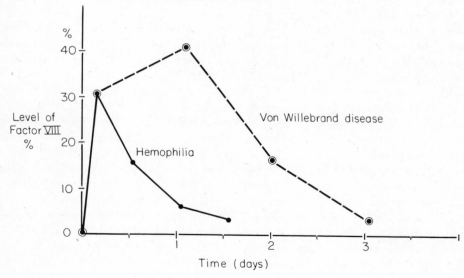

TABLE 18-2.—APPROXIMATE TURNOVER DATA ON COAGULATION FACTORS

FACTOR	PLASMA CONCENTRATION (μG/ML)	T$\frac{1}{2}$ (HR)	TURNOVER (μG/ML/24 HR)
I (Fibrinogen)	3000.0	100	600
II (Prothrombin)	150.0	72	50
V	50.0	16	15
VII	0.5	6	2
VIII (Antihemophilic)	10.0	12	20
IX (PTC)	3.0	24	3
X	15.0	48	7
XI (PTA)	?	60	?
XII (Hageman)	29.0	60	12
XIII (Fibrin-stabilizing)	20.0	120	4

surgery, are usually effective in producing normal hemostasis for dental extraction. Sockets of extracted teeth should not be sealed with sutures. The use of epsilon-amino caproic acid (350 mg/kg/day, orally for 7 days) with dental extraction may greatly reduce the transfusion requirement for factor VIII. About 5% of patients have factor VIII inhibitors and are resistant to infusions of factor VIII.

Physiotherapy is important following intra-articular bleeding, and follow-up management by orthopedic surgeons and physiotherapists is useful in avoiding later reparative surgery. Full weight-bearing should not be resumed until muscle power has been recovered. Patients with recurrent joint bleeding are greatly aided by physiotherapy. Temporary splinting may be required to prevent deformities.

18.1.1.5 COURSE AND PROGNOSIS.—Severe hemophiliacs manifest recurrent bleeding, which causes a variable degree of incapacity. Most hemophiliacs are capable of permanent employment. Transfusion therapy has prolonged life considerably and has enabled many patients to continue working at normal occupations. It is possible to train the patient or his family to give infusions at home and thereby permit treatment to start at a very early stage of the bleeding and significantly reduce morbidity. Mild hemo-

philiacs usually have a normal life except that special management is required after injury and surgery.

18.1.2 VON WILLEBRAND'S DISEASE

18.1.2.1 CLINICAL FEATURES.—Von Willebrand's disease is a hereditary hemorrhagic disorder inherited as an autosomal dominant trait and characterized by a prolonged bleeding time associated with a factor VIII coagulant activity reduced to less than 50% of the normal level. In most patients the hemorrhagic diathesis is mild; symptoms include epistaxis, easy bruising in response to trauma, and troublesome bleeding for a few days after minor lacerations and tooth extractions. If the coagulation defect is unusually severe, prolonged wound bleeding and hemarthroses may occur.

18.1.2.2 DIAGNOSIS.—The diagnosis is based primarily on laboratory tests including the bleeding time and factor VIII coagulant activity. Unlike hemophilia, factor VIII antigenic activity is reduced parallel to the reduced coagulant activity. In addition, abnormal platelet function may be demonstrated by (1) decreased platelet trapping when whole blood is passed through a column of glass beads and (2) defective platelet aggregation in vitro in response to the antibiotic, ristocetin. Other tests of platelet function, including clot retraction and platelet aggregation in response to ADP, collagen, thrombin and norepinephrine, are normal. These unique manifestations of von Willebrand's disease depend upon a defective serum protein. This protein is required for normal platelet function and also influences factor VIII activity. Infusion of hemophilic plasma into a patient with von Willebrand's disease leads to a slow rise in circulating factor VIII activity in the von Willebrand patient (see Fig. 18–2). Therefore, it would seem, the factor that is defective in von Willebrand's disease is present in the plasma of patients with classic hemophilia.

18.1.2.3 TREATMENT.—Local measures, as in hemophilia, are used in the case of mild bleeding due to von Willebrand's disease. Transfusion of normal plasma has a sustained effect on the factor VIII level, unlike the brief elevation in hemophilia. Cryoprecipitate also may be used in the therapy of von Willebrand's disease and produces a prolonged increase in factor VIII activity and improvement in hemostasis.

18.1.3 FACTOR IX (PLASMA THROMBOPLASTIN COMPONENT, PTC) DEFICIENCY

The incidence of factor IX deficiency is about 15% that of factor VIII deficiency. The clinical manifestations and inheritance are exactly as in hemophilia, but a different protein is defective and a different concentrate is used in therapy. As in factor VIII deficiency, it appears that most patients with factor IX deficiency actually synthesize a factor IX-like protein that has defective coagulant activity. Several different types of factor IX molecule with different degrees of coagulant activity have been described.

Factor IX concentrates are used in the treatment of factor IX deficiency. Infused factor IX has a half-life of 24 hours. Only 50% of the infused factor activity is recovered in the recipient's blood.

18.1.4 FACTOR XI (PLASMA THROMBOPLASTIN ANTECEDENT, PTA) DEFICIENCY

Clinically, factor XI deficiency resembles mild-to-moderate hemophilia. It is even less common than factor IX deficiency. A significant percentage of affected individuals appear to have no excessive bleeding at all. The disorder is transmitted as an autosomal dominant characteristic, and most cases have occurred in people of Jewish origin. The disorder is readily treated with infusions of fresh frozen plasma, the infused factor XI activity having an in vivo half-life of 60 hours.

18.1.5 FACTOR XII (HAGEMAN) DEFICIENCY

This deficiency usually is asymptomatic. The whole blood clotting time and partial thromboplastin time tests are grossly prolonged. The explanation for the lack of hemorrhagic diathesis is unknown. Two hypotheses have been proposed: (1) compensation by the extrinsic pathway and platelets for defective initiation of the intrinsic pathway, and (2) specific bypass of factor XII by direct activation of factor XI. Neither hypothesis is supported by convincing data.

18.1.6 FACTOR XIII (FIBRIN-STABILIZING) DEFICIENCY

Deficiency of factor XIII presents with a moderately severe bleeding tendency. Fibrin clots formed in this disorder fail to become cross-linked and are extremely susceptible to dissolution by plasmin. Excessive bleeding from the umbilicus and production of keloid scar tissue (often on the forehead) following bleeding from injury are suggestive of the disorder. The diagnostic test for factor XIII deficiency is dissolution of the clot formed from the patient's blood in 5 molar urea or trichloracetic acid. There are other causes of abnormal clot solubility and the diagnosis should be confirmed by a quantitative assay of factor XIII activity. All other coagulation tests are normal in this disorder. Transfusion with plasma temporarily restores normal hemostasis.

18.2 Acquired Coagulation Disorders

These disorders occur significantly more often than do the congenital disorders. They constitute the bulk of coagulation disorders encountered in a medical practice.

18.2.1 VITAMIN K DEFICIENCY

Vitamin K is a fat-soluble vitamin essential for the hepatic synthesis of prothrombin and factors VII, IX and X. Recent work has identified a newly identified amino acid, γ-carboxylic glutamic acid, in the normal prothrombin molecule. Prothrombin synthesized in the absence of vitamin K has glutamic acid in place of the γ-carboxylic glutamic acid. This biochemical abnormality is believed to be responsible for the deficient activity of prothrombin, and it is likely that a similar abnormality is responsible for the defective activity of factors VII, IX and X. These four coagulation factors are frequently referred to as the vitamin K-dependent coagulation factors. The sources of vitamin K are food and intestinal bacterial flora. The principal food sources of vitamin K are green leafy vegetables. There are relatively small body stores of vitamin K; if intake of vitamin K is stopped, deficiency may develop within 1–3 weeks. The diagnosis of vitamin K deficiency is confirmed if a prolonged one-stage prothrombin time test is corrected in 12–24 hours by parenteral administration of vitamin K.

18.2.1.1 CAUSES.—Vitamin K deficiency may arise by a number of different mechanisms. Impaired absorption of vitamin K due to lack of bile salts may result from obstruc-

tive jaundice and biliary fistula. Malabsorption due to idiopathic steatorrhea and other causes also can result in vitamin K deficiency. Alteration of the intestinal bacterial flora by antibiotics produces vitamin K deficiency by loss of that vitamin K synthesized by the normal flora. Hemorrhagic disease of the newborn has a complex pathogenesis including contributions from functional immaturity of the liver, a degree of vitamin K deficiency and inadequate gut flora.

18.2.1.2 TREATMENT.—Proper therapy must involve correction of the underlying cause. Vitamin K, which will immediately correct the defect, can be administered either as the naturally occurring oil-soluble vitamin K_1 or as a synthetic vitamin K. Preparations of vitamin K_1 include both oral and intravenous forms. Vitamin K_1 is the most potent and rapidly acting form, correcting coagulation abnormalities within 6–12 hours of intravenous administration. Vitamin K_1 should be used for treatment of hemorrhagic disease in the newborn or for any vitamin K deficiency if bleeding is active. Oral and parenteral preparations of synthetic vitamin K also are available. These synthetic preparations may be used for treatment in the absence of bleeding and for maintenance vitamin K replacement. They should not be used in the neonate, since they may cause hemolysis and kernicterus in infants with G-6-PD deficiency. Response to therapy always should be confirmed by repeating the prothrombin time 24 hours after administration of vitamin K. Failure to correct the prothrombin time signifies failure to absorb the vitamin K or liver disease. If more urgent correction of the hemostatic defect is required than can be provided by administration of vitamin K, plasma or a concentrate of the vitamin K-dependent factors may be infused.

18.2.2 ANTICOAGULANT DRUGS

Commonly used anticoagulant drugs include the dicoumarol derivatives and heparin. *Dicoumarol* acts by antagonizing the action of vitamin K and leads to the same clotting abnormalities as does vitamin K deficiency. The effects of dicoumarol include a long prothrombin time and partial thromboplastin time and reduced levels of prothrombin and factors VII, IX and X. Abnormal bleeding is the chief complication of overdosage, which may be due to error, accident or attempted suicide. The drugs usually implicated are dicoumarol (half-life, 24 hours) and warfarin (half-life, 40 hours). Treatment consists of vitamin K administration and infusion of plasma or a coagulation factor concentrate, if bleeding is severe.

The best known action of *heparin* is the inactivation of thrombin, which prevents thrombin from acting on fibrinogen. In a purified system heparin does not inactivate thrombin. In blood heparin binds to a lysine side chain on the antithrombin molecule and thereby greatly accelerates a stoichiometric reaction between thrombin and antithrombin, which results in inactivation of thrombin. Heparin also acts earlier in the coagulation sequence, inactivating factors Xa, IXa and XIa by accelerating formation of inactive complexes with antithrombin. An average dose of heparin is cleared from the blood in about 6 hours. The principal clearance mechanisms are excretion by the urine and inactivation by a liver heparinase. All coagulation tests are affected by heparin including the one-stage prothrombin time. The most sensitive tests, usually used to monitor the pharmacologic effect of heparin, are the whole blood clotting time, partial thromboplastin time and thrombin time.

Treatment of bleeding associated with excessive heparin is relatively simple. Heparin is a strongly negatively charged molecule and can be rapidly neutralized, milligram for milligram, by intravenous administration of protamine sulfate, which is strongly positively charged. Before infusing protamine, the amount of protamine required to neutralize the circulating heparin can be determined in vitro by a protamine titration test.

18.2.3 Liver Disease

Liver disease is one of the commonest causes of bleeding disorder and is very difficult to treat. The principal disorders of function appear to be decreased protein synthesis, due to liver cell failure, and increased proteolytic activity, perhaps due to decrease in the liver's capacity to remove active enzymes from the circulating blood. Increased fibrinolytic activity is consistently present in instances of cirrhosis and liver failure. There is some evidence that intravascular coagulation (see section 18.2.5) also may occur in liver failure, but the contribution of this mechanism has not been adequately defined. The net effect of these pathologic changes is to reduce the levels of all coagulation factors except that of factor VIII. The hemostatic defect is commonly compounded by thrombocytopenia as well.

In severe liver disease a common pattern of hemostatic abnormalities includes a low fibrinogen level, long prothrombin time and normal or long partial thromboplastin time. The normal partial thromboplastin time may be the result of an elevated factor VIII level, which can compensate for low levels of the other factors. The reason for the increased factor VIII concentration is not known. The thrombin time usually is prolonged, but the mechanism also is not clear. Heparin infusions may transiently elevate the fibrinogen level, suggesting that the low fibrinogen level may be due in part to catabolism from thrombin-mediated proteolysis. Heparin seldom restores the fibrinogen level to normal. The effect of heparin on clinical hemostasis is variable; oozing may transiently diminish but is apt to be followed by increased bleeding due to the anticoagulant effect of heparin. Fibrinolytic inhibitors appear to have at best a transiently beneficial effect. In the management of frank bleeding, infusion of plasma may be preferable to infusion of coagulation factor concentrates. Some concentrates contain active coagulation enzymes, which, being poorly cleared by the failing liver, can aggravate intravascular clotting and compound the problem. In general, bleeding due to liver failure is very difficult to treat unless improvement in liver cell function occurs.

18.2.4 FIBRINOGEN DEFICIENCY

The normal plasma concentration of fibrinogen varies between 200 and 400 mg/100 ml. Elevated levels occur during pregnancy and during acute febrile reactions. Deficiency of fibrinogen may be congenital or acquired.

18.2.4.1 CONGENITAL DEFICIENCY OF FIBRINOGEN. — This may manifest as a complete or partial absence of fibrinogen from the blood plasma. The disorder is transmitted as an autosomal recessive trait. Clinically the disease resembles moderate or mild hemophilia except for absence of hemarthroses. When there is complete absence of fibrinogen, the whole blood clotting time, one-stage prothrombin time and thrombin clotting time all are grossly prolonged. Control of bleeding is achieved by transfusion of fibrinogen or freshly frozen plasma. With partial deficiencies of fibrinogen, of the order of 25 – 50 mg/100 ml, the screening coagulation tests may show only minor abnormality, and only a quantitative measure of the fibrinogen level indicates the presence of a deficiency.

Another class of congenital fibrinogen abnormality is due to the hereditary synthesis of structurally and functionally abnormal fibrinogen molecules, a situation analogous to some of the hemoglobinopathies. Fibrinogen Detroit has an amino acid substitution, serine for arginine, at position 19 on the $A\alpha$ polypeptide chain. The propositus presented with grossly excessive bleeding. Over a dozen additional patients with molecular abnormalities of fibrinogen have been identified, although the biochemical defect has not been established in each case. Some of these patients display a severe hemorrhagic syndrome; others are asymptomatic. The laboratory finding most useful in identifying these

abnormalities is a prolonged thrombin clotting time.

18.2.4.2 ACQUIRED DEFICIENCY OF FIBRINOGEN. — This may be due to impaired synthesis or accelerated destruction of the protein. Impaired synthesis is seen in hepatitis, in hepatic necrosis and following administration of L-asparaginase in treatment of leukemia. Accelerated destruction usually results from increased blood proteolytic activity. The commonest causes of increased proteolytic activity are discussed in the next section.

18.2.5 DISSEMINATED INTRAVASCULAR COAGULATION

Several terms have been used to describe the clinical syndrome characterized by acquired hypofibrinogenemia due to excessively rapid utilization of fibrinogen. These include the defibrination syndrome, DIC and consumption coagulopathy.

18.2.5.1 CLINICAL FEATURES. — There are both acute and subacute variants of DIC, which are distinguished by the rapidity of onset and severity of symptoms.

The *acute* form is associated with a number of clinical conditions, including:

1. Complications of pregnancy: premature separation of the placenta and amniotic fluid embolism.

2. Overwhelming sepsis and shock, the latter being the principal factor. Infections implicated are most often due to gram-negative organisms, especially meningococci; DIC in conjunction with infection by gram-positive organisms, viruses, rickettsiae and malarial parasites has been reported.

3. Shock from any cause, including hemorrhagic shock and shock associated with cardiac arrest.

4. Incompatible blood transfusion.

5. Acute, vigorous hemolysis.

6. Surgery, especially on lungs or liver.

7. Anaphylaxis.

8. Heat stroke or burn.

9. Snake bite, especially by the Malayan pit viper.

10. Rejection of transplanted organs.

11. Purpura fulminans, a form of purpura chiefly affecting children, characterized by sudden onset of fever, prostration and cutaneous ecchymoses that extend rapidly and may become gangrenous.

Subacute DIC is found in association with the following:

1. Intrauterine retention of a dead fetus in the later stages of pregnancy.

2. Neoplastic disease, usually when metastases are present. Neoplasms most frequently associated are carcinoma of the prostate, pancreas and lung.

3. Leukemia, especially the promyelocytic, acute myeloblastic and acute lymphatic varieties.

4. SLE.

5. Cavernous hemangioma (Kasabach-Merritt syndrome).

6. Liver failure. The contribution of DIC to the hemostatic defect in liver failure is not yet established.

18.2.5.2 LABORATORY STUDIES.—The cardinal laboratory sign of the syndrome is an altered fibrinogen level or evidence of proteolytic attack on the fibrinogen molecule. The normal fibrinogen level is 200–400 mg/100 ml. Levels of under 100 mg/100 ml are unequivocally low. Since the patient's normal fibrinogen level is rarely known, a fibrinogen level within the normal range cannot be accepted as unequivocal evidence against DIC. Two useful tests for qualitative alterations in circulating fibrinogen are the thrombin time and tests for fibrinogen/fibrin degradation products (FDP). The thrombin time is one of the simplest and most rapidly performed tests, but it also is affected by the presence of heparin, some dysproteinemias and congenital dysfibrinogenemia.

Other coagulation tests may be abnormal in DIC, due largely to consumption of coagulation factors by thrombin and plasmin. The prothrombin time may be prolonged due to reduced factor V concentration. The partial thromboplastin time may be prolonged due to decreased factor VIII. Factor V and VIII assay levels are usually but not always low. Thrombocytopenia of some degree is almost invariable. Assays for plasma fibrinolytic activity, e.g., the euglobulin lysis test, give variable results.

18.2.5.3 PATHOGENESIS.—Despite extensive investigation, the pathogenesis of the disorder remains incompletely understood. A possible hypothesis to explain the clinical findings is that two active enzymes—thrombin and plasmin—are formed in the circulating blood. Thrombin coagulates fibrinogen, forming clots and reducing the blood fibrinogen concentration. At low concentration, thrombin activates factors V and VIII; at high concentration, thrombin destroys the activity of these two coagulation factors. Thrombin also triggers platelet aggregation, causing thrombocytopenia. Plasmin (fibrinolysin) digests both fibrinogen and fibrin, forming FDP. These *FDP* act as anticoagulants at the stage of thrombin action on fibrinogen; they inhibit the normal orderly polymerization of fibrin and also inhibit the normal functioning of platelets in an as yet undefined manner. Plasmin also digests and inactivates factors V and VIII. Plasmin does not aggregate platelets or cause thrombocytopenia. It is postulated that, as a consequence of these complex enzymatic effects, a generalized bleeding tendency may develop.

18.2.5.4 MANAGEMENT.—The principal goal in management is treatment of the primary disease. If this is successfully accomplished, the coagulation abnormality will in time be corrected. The presence of shock is the major factor determining mortality rate and must be corrected as rapidly as possible. The coagulation abnormalities can be treated with anticoagulants and specific factor infusions if a clear diagnosis of DIC has been established, if overt bleeding is present and if time is needed for correction of the primary disorder. Heparin can be used to interrupt the coagulation process and prevent further consumption of hemostatic factors, but the exact role of the heparin in therapy of DIC has not been determined. Replacement of deficient hemostatic factors should be begun together with heparin administration. Freshly frozen plasma will replace factor V and VIII activity, and platelet concentrates can be administered for severe thrombocytopenia.

18.2.6 CIRCULATING ANTICOAGULANTS

Most naturally occurring circulating anticoagulants are actually antibodies to specific clotting factors. Patients have been described with antibodies to fibrinogen and factors V, VIII, IX, X, XI and XIII. Antibodies may arise in patients with congenitally deficient factor activity or in patients with a previously normal coagulation system. In the latter case, the antibody may be an isolated finding or may be only part of a complex autoimmune syndrome such as SLE.

18.2.6.1 CLINICAL AND LABORATORY FEATURES. — The clinical manifestations of an antibody-type circulating anticoagulant are similar to congenital deficiency of the affected factor. The principal difference is that replacement therapy is generally ineffective, and steroid therapy is ineffective unless the primary disease (e.g., SLE) is steroid responsive. The disorder may persist indefinitely or may remit spontaneously and unpredictably.

Laboratory studies reveal all the features of deficiency of the specific factor. For example, if the antibody is to factor VIII, there is a long partial thromboplastin time, low factor VIII level and normal prothrombin time. Furthermore, the patient's plasma induces a factor VIII deficiency in normal plasma when the two are mixed. The patient's plasma also will inactivate purified factor VIII in a time-dependent reaction. Antibodies to factor VIII are the most common antibodies encountered: they occur in about 5% of hemophiliacs transiently and rarely in postpartum women; in association with penicillin allergy; in patients with SLE and rheumatoid arthritis and at times without apparent cause. Despite poor laboratory evidence of an increase in specific level, infusion of the appropriate concentrate may be life saving.

18.2.6.2 SYSTEMIC LUPUS ERYTHEMATOSUS. — In addition to the circulating antibody anticoagulants already described, patients with SLE may develop antibody directed against prothrombin activator, the hemostatic factor responsible for *prothrombin conversion* to thrombin. Clinically, there usually is little or no excessive bleeding other than bruising. Thrombophlebitis has been reported in some patients. Laboratory features of the disorder include a prolonged whole blood clotting time, prothrombin time and partial thromboplastin time. The patient's prothrombin level is low. Other factor assays are normal. A mixture of patient's and normal plasma has a long prothrombin time and partial thromboplastin time. This condition usually responds rapidly to steroid therapy, often with return to normal of the coagulation findings within a week. However, the coagulation findings themselves are not an indication for steroid therapy, which should be used as described for the underlying disease.

RECOMMENDED READING

ATLASES:

Hayhoe, F. G. J., and Flemans, R. J.: *An Atlas of Haematological Cytology* (New York: John Wiley & Sons, Inc., 1970).

Sandoz Atlas of Haematology (2d ed.; Hanover, N. J.: Sandoz Pharmaceuticals, 1973).

GENERAL TEXTS:

Cartwright, G. E.: *Diagnostic Laboratory Hematology* (4th ed.; New York: Grune & Stratton, 1968).

Hardesty, R. M., and Weatherall, D. J.: *Blood and Its Disorders* (Oxford: Blackwell Scientific Publications, 1974).

Williams, W. J., Beutler, E., Erslev, A. J., and Rundles, W. R.: *Hematology* (New York: McGraw-Hill Book Co., 1972).

Wintrobe, M. M., Lee, R. G., Boggs, D. R., Bithell, T. C., Athens, J. W., and Foerster, J.: *Clinical Hematology* (7th ed.; Philadelphia: Lea & Febiger, 1974).

PERIODICALS:

Blood (Grune & Stratton; monthly).

British Journal of Haematology (Blackwell Scientific Publications; monthly).

Progress in Hematology (Grune & Stratton; approximately biennially).

Seminars in Hematology (Grune & Stratton; quarterly).

Appendix:
Normal Values for Hematologic Tests

(If not otherwise indicated, these are mean values for adults ± s.d. The asterisk indicates values in children. Newborn values are for day 1 of life. All values are subject to some variation depending on geographic region and specific laboratory.)

Parameter	Abbreviation	Value	Unit
Red blood cell count	RBC		
Men		0.5 ± 0.4	$\times 10^6/\mu l$ blood
Women		4.5 ± 0.4	same
Newborn		5.8 ± 0.4	same
Hemoglobin	Hb		
Men		15.5 ± 1	gm/100 ml blood
Women		14.0 ± 1	same
Newborn		18.0 ± 1	same
Hematocrit	Hct		
Men		46.0 ± 3	ml/100 ml blood
Women		41.0 ± 3	same
Newborn		58.0 ± 3	same
White blood cell count	WBC		
Adult		7.25 ± 1.85	$\times 10^3/\mu l$ blood
Newborn		12.2 ± 2.00	same
Differential leukocyte count			
Neutrophils—Total	Neut.	59(50*)	%
segmented		56(47*)	%
bands		3(3*)	%
Eosinophils	Eos.	3(2*)	%
Basophils	Baso.	1(1*)	%
Lymphocytes	Lymph.	33(42*)	%
Monocytes	Mono.	4(5*)	%
Platelet count	Plts.		
Adult		300 ± 100	$\times 10^3/\mu l$ blood
Newborn		190 ± 50	same

151

Mean corpuscular volume	MCV	90 ± 5	μm^3/red cell
Mean corpuscular hemoglobin	MCH	30 ± 2	pg/red cell
Mean corpuscular hemoglobin concentration	MCHC	33.7 ± 1.1	gm/100 ml RBC
Reticulocytes	Retic.	$0-1$	%
Blood volume	B.V.		
Men		69	ml/kg
Women		65	ml/kg
Red cell mass			
Men		$25-32$	ml/kg
Women		$23-30$	same
Plasma volume	P.V.		
Men		39	ml/kg
Women		40	same
Serum iron	Ser Fe	$80-160$	μg/100 ml
Total iron-binding capacity	TIBC	$250-400$	μg/100 ml
Transferrin		$1-2$	gm/1
Serum haptoglobin		$0.3-2$	gm/1
Hemoglobin A_2	HbA_2	2.5 ± 0.5	%
Fetal hemoglobin	HbF		
Adult		2 ± 0.5	%
Newborn		$65-90$	%
Red cell life span ^{51}chromium	^{51}Cr RBC t$^{1/2}$	$25-32$	days
Serum folate	Ser F.A.	$6-20$	μg/ml
Serum vitamin B_{12}	Ser vit B_{12}	$150-600$	pg/ml
Bilirubin			
Unconjugated		<0.2	mg/100 ml
Conjugated		<0.6	mg/100 ml
Prothrombin time	PT	12	sec
Bleeding time (IV technic)		<6	min
Whole blood clotting time (Lee-White)	CT	$4-8$	min
Fibrinogen		$200-400$	mg/100 ml
Partial thromboplastin time	PTT	$55-65$	sec
Activated PTT	APTT	$35-40$	sec

Index